101 Top Tips in Medicine

D0303124

101 Top Tips in Medicine

CYNICAL AND OTHERWISE

JOHN LARKIN

Radcliffe Publishing
Oxford • New York

Radcliffe Publishing Ltd
18 Marcham Road
Abingdon
Oxon OX14 1AA
United Kingdom

www.radcliffe-oxford.com
Electronic catalogue and worldwide online ordering facility.

British Library Cataloguing in Publication Data

A catalogue record for this book is available from the British Library.

ISBN-13: 978 184619 398 9

The paper used for the text pages of this book
is FSC certified. FSC (The Forest Stewardship
Council) is an international network to promote
responsible management of the world's forests.

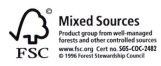

Mixed Sources
Product group from well-managed
forests and other controlled sources
www.fsc.org Cert no. SGS-COC-2482
© 1996 Forest Stewardship Council

Typeset by Pindar NZ, Auckland, New Zealand
Printed and bound by TJI Digital, Padstow, Cornwall, UK

Contents

To Peter, Anna and Catherine.

About the author

John Larkin was brought up in Lanarkshire and trained at the University of Glasgow. Early days in rheumatology were followed by some dabbling in diabetes and clinical pharmacology (to the tune of his MD thesis) before returning to his 'first love'. His positions as Honorary Clinical Senior Lecturer and (often reluctant) Examiner for the College sit uneasily on inherently frivolous shoulders. Teaching should still be 'a bit of fun, Dougal'. He is married with three adult offspring. He remains exceedingly grumpy.

Acknowledgements

My thanks are due to Fiona McGarry who reviewed the cynical tips for insufficient cynicism, and Howard McAlpine who scanned all the others for insufficient accuracy. The numerous expected complaints should thus be sent to them directly. Appreciation is also due to those who supplied individual tips (*see* 'Culprits'), as well as to the juniors and patients who inspired both theirs and my own. Finally thanks to all at Radcliffe, for their kind opinions on the Emperor's latest pair of jeans.

Introduction

All right. Let's come clean. These aren't really *the* top 101 medical tips.

First of all, there's no way my clinical-tip-number-seven is going to be as important as *'when auscultating, always use your stethoscope'*, or *'always examine the abdomen with the patient lying down'*, or even *'never perform fundoscopy with a pencil tucked behind your ear'*. But there would be little point in stuffing a book full of self-evident half-truths. Indeed, you could argue that such pieces of advice are not 'tips' in the first place. The word 'Tip' suggests something that is not widely recognised, something a bit 'off the wall'. A stable lad doesn't ring up the local bookie at three in the morning with a 'tip' that the odds-on favourite is going to win tomorrow's big Handicap. Tips should carry some novelty value, and arguably some uncertainty. Perhaps even danger. Tips are basically personal opinions, and as such run the risk of being entirely inaccurate – in the case of my own tips, a quite substantial risk. You just gotta suck-it-and-see.

Second of all, these can't even be *my* top 101 tips, since to do that I'd have to repeat all my best tips from all my previous books (OK . . . one . . .). So the plan was to go to all of my colleagues (senior and not-so-senior), get half a dozen top tips from each of them and write them up in my own fortunately inimitable style – each tip's original author being appropriately acknowledged. Fifteen months into this plan, they had collectively produced the princely sum of two pearls of wisdom – *always keep your medical insurance up-to-date*, and *don't write tip books*.

The upshot of which was my setting off on a single-handed voyage on the stormy seas of tipdom – prompting a few genuine suggestions from hitherto silent quarters which have been incorporated and attributed using initials.

There may or may not be a list of these initials and their owners at the end of the book, depending on space, publisher's whim and the willingness of those initials to be associated with a publication which will at best teeter on the edge of respectability.

Indeed, this dearth of *bon mots* from my lazy colleagues resulted in a superfluity of such teetering. Initial high-quality tips gave way to personal rants about various bees-in-my-bonnet. Most, I now realise, have been prompted by disparate occurrences in the clinic, on the wards and at the teaching bedside. I suppose I must feel sorry for the various juniors obliged to feign interest at any of my 'Eureka' moments, though one bright spark did throw my phraseology back at me when he came to my office for some case notes. He looked around the untidy morass of case sheets and papers and books and pamphlets and chess pieces and elastic bands (I'm busy!) and commented, 'You could use *this* as a tip'.

Cynical Tips

The ideology behind cynical acumen is, if not pure, certainly simple. If we are to help the patient in front of us to the best of our ability, then it seems self-evident that we should start off by making the correct diagnosis. Not the diagnosis they think they've got or the one they want to have. Not the diagnosis their family or friends think they've got or the one they want them to have. Not even the diagnosis that some other doctor thinks or says they have. Just the real one.

Put like that, the whole thing doesn't sound particularly cynical, indeed might appear entirely laudable. But it's the inherent presumption that all those other diagnoses might be 'wrong', and the implication that there may be underlying reasons for this, that bring the double-edged qualities of 'cynicism' to our approach – and with them some semblance of disrepute. Plus, of course, the techniques you have to use to elicit the true diagnosis.

These techniques might themselves be summed up in a single concept. Be aware of the things that you know, but the patient doesn't know – and use them. It's always amazed me when TV detectives interview a suspect, almost inevitably displaying total disregard for this principle. You know the sort of thing:

> So, Mr Blenkinsop, where were you last night at eight thirty? – and don't tell us you were at the opera because last night's performance was cancelled, and don't say you were at home all night because we have a witness who saw you leaving a twenty-four-hour grocery store at twelve twenty-six . . .

Thus giving Blenkinsop ample warning and a few vital seconds to come up with a reasonable story. If he's particularly clever, he won't quite start his answer with '*Mmmm . . . in that case . . . I was at . . .*'

Why don't they just ask the questions blind, and get the patient's – sorry – *suspect*'s first answers? Then when they are clearly incompatible with something the policeman already knows – well, that tells you something, doesn't it?

So.

Since my approach to the doctor–patient relationship is the entirely reprehensible one of seeing myself as an Inspector Morse to the patient's devious serial killer, I obviously want to avoid making the same mistake as the cops. Keep my powder dry, as it were.

Don't let them know what *you* know until you got 'em bang to rights . . . Guv . . .

CYNICAL TIP 1: PRESS THE SPINOUS PROCESSES

We'll start with a nice example of using something you – as a medical practitioner – know, but which the patient does not. Which is that nothing (well, almost nothing[1]) actually makes the spinous processes tender. Particularly helpful as most lay-people assume that anything causing major back pain must also make it sore to touch. So if you think the patient is overdoing the extent of their back pain – and the traditional straight-leg-raising-to-30°-is-painful-in-someone-who-can-sit-bolt-upright-with-their-legs-stretched-in-front-of-them doesn't clarify things – then a gratuitous pressing of all the vertebral processes is called for. If any more than one of these is any more than marginally tender then the patient is overplaying their hand (patients with three genuinely slipped discs will find it 'no problem').

It's worth noting that this is indeed an entirely 'gratuitous' test since the genuine causes of such tenderness (osteomyelitis . . . er . . . maybe tumour . . . more osteomyelitis) are so rare as to render the manoeuvre almost useless to the non-cynical practitioner in a normal clinic. You will, however, see such practitioners (and there's a lot of them out there) do it. Don't stop them. They're what makes it work for us guys.

The test is most effective when the patient finds all or nearly all the

---

1   It's a well-known medical tenet that you should never say 'never', well, almost never.

processes excruciatingly painful when gently pressed – an unlikely finding that is surprisingly common. Indeed, it is worth trying the test in patients with any rheumatological complaints (not just back pain) that don't ring true. They'll often claim spinous process tenderness just to crank up the severity of their problems a notch.

CYNICAL TIP 2: PAY NO ATTENTION TO A FAMILY HISTORY OF RHEUMATOID ARTHRITIS

You'd never believe the sort of referral letters I get from GPs.

> Dear Dr
> This 45-year-old woman has a 15-year history of aches and pains in all of her joints. There's no morning exacerbation, examination is entirely normal, blood tests are all normal including a negative Rheumatoid Factor. X-rays show nothing untoward. There doesn't seem to be any inflammatory arthropathy, but her mother had RA so I wonder if you could see her at the rheumatology clinic as an urgency.

Why?

The GP has already done all the right things, and there's no suggestion this woman has rheumatoid arthritis.

You don't make a diagnosis based on the family history. You make it on the symptoms, the signs and the results.[2] The GP might as well finish 'but her mother had fibroids' and then send her to the gynaecologist.

I think the problem boils down to a misconception of why we take a family history. It doesn't clinch a diagnosis. If someone might have either RA or OA, you don't decide it's OA 'cos that's the one they have in the family. I have seen people make a similar mistake using 'epidemiology' – deciding that a man with clear rheumatoid arthritis has ankylosing spondylitis 'because he's a man and "ank spond" is commoner in males.'

Makes no sense.

We take a family history to alert us to anything in there that otherwise we might not have considered. Rare things. So if the patient's parents had Familial Mediterranean fever, or sickle-cell anaemia, or even tuberculosis two months ago – then that's worth knowing. But it doesn't differentiate between

---

2   If it doesn't walk like a duck, or swim like a duck, or quack like a duck, then it isn't a duck – even if its mother was a d- . . . OK. Bad analogy.

two possible diagnoses. It's the same with the trendy use of family history as part of the assessment of risk factors, e.g. for ischaemic heart disease. So it might point us towards starting someone with a borderline cholesterol on a statin. What it doesn't do is affect our diagnosis – make us decide that a man with sharp left-sided chest pain, worse on inspiration, with a cough and green spit has actually had a myocardial infarction because that's what his dad had.

The plethora of patients at our clinic with a family history of rheumatoid and a personal history of nothing-like-rheumatoid actually prompted me to 'research' this phenomenon in a year's worth of patients. We found that a family history of RA was a statistically significantly better predictor of NOT having RA than of having RA.[3] Of course there is some heritability to RA, but it looked like the effect of a positive family history[4] on the psyches of the patient and their GP had more to do with their eventual attendance at my clinic than any increase in the incidence of actual arthritis.

Which all means, I suppose, that there might be *some* merit in taking the family history. If someone clearly has **Nothing-Wrong-With-Them** (NoWWT [*vide* much *infra*]) at the clinic, then realising their worries are based on a family history might argue against the necessity of digging deeper for psychological or other reasons for them being there in the first place.

Just don't think that it means they've got RA.

---

3   Though not *per se* a statistically significant predictor of NOT having RA. That would have been too brilliant. Budding statisticians among you will recognise the difference, but deny its existence.

4   Or what they think is a family history of RA. Most people remember the words *rheumatoid arthritis* but not the word *osteoarthritis* (there's *osteoporosis* to confuse it with, for a start). So any vague arthritis somebody had in the past will be called 'rheumatoid' just to keep the conversation going.

CYNICAL TIP 3: DON'T TELL THE PATIENT WHAT YOU'RE EXAMINING UNLESS IT'S ABSOLUTELY NECESSARY

A problem.

This tip would fit into any of the four categories. Indeed I considered including it in all four, leapfrogging myself towards the magical '101' tips. But Sloth is a seductive and dangerous path to tread. (*Clinical Tip 4: How to take a tricky blood pressure . . . this time in the* **left** *arm . . .*)

So which category?

Clinical-wise it's often useful to keep your target from the patient. Not doing so may a) affect the result, or b) affect your ability to achieve the result.

We all know that if the patient is aware we are counting his breathing, this will influence our findings. The same is probably true of the pulse, and if we could engineer a way to sneak up behind him and take the BP without his knowing, we'd jump at it[5] (though probably thus losing the element of surprise).

Alternatively, if you let him know you're looking for a neck vein, he'll helpfully stretch his head into an extremely unhelpful position, plus breathe in hugely when you press on the abdomen (don't tell him you're about to![6]), reducing intra-thoracic pressure and totally negating your desired effect of increasing the JVP. Even the simple ploy of asking him to breathe through his mouth will immediately induce spectacular nose-breathing – particularly in men of a certain age.[7]

So don't mention anything, unless it's of its nature tricky to explain retrospectively ('calm down a minute . . . so why did you **think** I was putting a latex glove on? . . .').

Career-wise, while in an exam, there seems to me little point telling the patient you're going to examine his spleen and then doing all the right things to examine . . . his liver, when if you'd kept your mouth shut the dopey examiner would never have spotted anything amiss, and assumed you were competently examining for the organ you intended.

Survival-wise, if you're going to go around telling every patient what you're examining then you'll spend your life explaining why you did that, why you're doing this, how the examination works, why it is that your way of

5 Nearest equivalent is continual monitoring of BP via machine – which confirms the expected drop in BP as the patient gets used to it.
6 But don't hurt him.
7 Which, I realise, is why I have assumed throughout that this patient is male.

doing it is totally different from all the other doctors (including the professor!) who've examined for the same thing . . . and what did you find? . . . is it big? . . . is that good? . . . is that bad? . . . seriously bad? . . . seriously good? . . . But when all's said and done, there is only one place for this tip to find a home.

It's a **Cynical** Tip, through and through.

When confronted by the dubious patient, it's extremely important that you do not tell them exactly what your examination manoeuvre is designed to test. That way they'll be forced to guess what it's testing, react in the fashion they expect their hypothetical illness would make them react to this completely other test, and will hopefully fall flat on their faces (metaphorically speaking, of course[8]).

Not revealing the purpose of examination is, of course, only useful in certain circumstances. There is little point in hiding the fact we are listening for mitral stenosis in the hope that the patient will give themselves away by feigning the murmur of aortic incompetence. Indeed, as with most cynical tips, we find few situations in the examination of heart, lungs or abdomen where it comes in useful. The locomotor and neurological systems, on the other hand, are much more dependent on the patient's subjective response ('is this painful?' . . . 'can you feel that?' . . . 'can you push as hard as you can?' . . . 'does that feel fuzzy or normal?' . . . 'no, no – what do *you* mean by "fuzzy"?'). And here, not allowing the patient the luxury of knowing exactly what's going on comes into its own.

RHEUMATOLOGY (STARTING FROM HANDS AND WORKING . . . INWARDS)

Don't tell patient why you are pressing their MCPs and PIPs. Trust me. Most punters feigning raging inflammatory arthritis won't realise this should be painful until it's too late.

Don't tell them why you're doing Tinel's and Phalen's tests. Just ask if they feel anything (subliminally suggesting that this might be pain rather than tingling). Certainly DON'T give away that any tingling should be in thumb and two-and-a-half fingers. Unprompted, most punters will opt for the pinkie.

---

8   It would be over-zealous cynicism to perform Romberg's test, and gleefully note that the patient erroneously fell flat on their face when a truly proprioceptively challenged person would have fallen to the side . . .

(Similar to this is the situation when you are taking a history from some-one who has 'volunteered' they have Carpal Tunnel Syndrome. They will say their fingers tingle and you first ask 'which fingers?' and when they say all of them you ask 'including the thumb?' and only once this is answered do you ask '. . . and what about the pinkie?' DO NOT GET THESE OUT OF ORDER. When you ask about a specific finger, the shrewd chancer will smell a rat, and may say it isn't affected, reverting to a 'yes' when asked about another finger. By asking in the above order, this shows them up as someone who clearly hasn't got Carpal Tunnel Syndrome and hasn't memorised the chapter well enough. But if you ask about the pinkie first, they'll escape the gallows.)[9,10]

When 'rotating the wrist' don't let on that this really rotates part of the elbow.

When getting them to flex and extend wrists ('make like you're revving up a motorbike, missus') against resistance, make no mention of tennis and golfer's elbow(s).[11] If they do spot that flicker of your eyes towards the elbow, fall back on the hope that the medial common origin (*flexor*) will get sore when patient is *extending* wrist and vice versa. And if you can't remember which one is golfer's elbow and which one is tennis elbow . . . join the club.

And there are lots of other things to not mention.

Left to the patient's own devices . . .

➤ Painful arc – most will describe pain during the wrong part of the arc (usually right at the top).
➤ Neck, lateral flexion – will cause pain on the side it moves towards . . . not usually the case.
➤ Hip – passive movements will cause pain in the knee.
➤ Hip rotation with knee bent (the most sensitive test for pain on hip movement) will also cause pain at the ankle, where you're holding it (at least, it does whenever I do this test . . . even in genuine patients . . . in fact, particularly in genuine patients . . . hmmm . . . might be doing something wrong).
➤ Knee – passive flexion will cause pain in middle of kneecap.
➤ Knee-to-contralateral-shoulder – will cause pain almost anywhere other than the sacroiliac joint which it stresses.

---

9   A bizarre full-paragraph-in-brackets. I've resolved to cut down on footnotes.
10   Damn!
11   Why isn't it a 'golf' elbow? Or alternatively a 'tennis player's elbow'?

NEUROLOGY

In general, cranial nerve examination doesn't lend itself to much mucking about on the patient's part – though I have had one patient with an unlikely hemiparesis decide he would spice it up with unilateral face involvement. An entertaining examination of cranial nerves ensued, with neither of us having any idea quite what would happen next.

Rinne's and Weber's testing are certainly best done with a certain fluidity, such that the patient has little opportunity to work out exactly what is happening (otherwise they might spot the paradoxical ear to hear 'Weber's' in).

Also worth not saying is what you expect to happen when checking the corneal reflex. Mind you, this is probably a clinical tip. I can see that the information (the eye should blink) could make someone with an absent reflex blink by some voluntary mechanism – but I'm not sure if all the contrary willpower in the world could get you to feign its absence.[12]

When performing the 'pronator drift' test – don't mention the words 'pronator drift' just in case the patient has medical knowledge and realises (despite the fact that 80% of doctors performing the manoeuvre don't) that an arm should not drift straight down if weak, but should drift slightly down whilst rotating outwards (towards pronation from initially supine position). Anything entirely straight should raise suspicion.

Oh yeah. Sex workers. Don't tell them why you're shining a light in their eyes, or they'll deliberately focus on the tip of their nose and you'll miss their Argyll Robertson pupils. Honest.

---

12 The corneal reflex is perhaps an apposite point to emphasise that while in all of these scenarios you don't tell the patient the purpose of your manoeuvre, you do mention the manoeuvre itself, i.e. that you're gonna poke their eye with an aggressive slice of cotton wool, or (my favoured style) romantically whisper sweet nothings across the corner of their cornea.

CYNICAL TIP 4: EXAMINE UPPER LIMB DERMATOMES FIRST-OFF IN THE NON-ANATOMICAL POSITION[13]

Another nice example of using knowledge the patient doesn't have. That neat dermatome map of the arms – revolving sweetly around the fulcrum of the C7-middle finger, with changes at the wrist and the elbow – is BAD NEWS for doctors. Because it makes sense. Total sense. Intuitively perfect. Any patient making up fuzzy areas might well fortuitously make up a couple that hang together anatomically. However . . . that perfect symmetry depends entirely on the arms being in the anatomical position . . . palms forward, arms held down at sides, slightly apart from body.

So.

Examine these dermatomes first-off with the arms in a very much non-anatomical position (my preference is flexed at the elbows and lightly held across the body). Any bogus anaesthesia or paraesthesia will almost certainly be in ridiculous juxtaposed areas (e.g. down the outer border of the arm onto the ulnar side of the forearm, i.e. C5 plus T1).

Personally I have to follow this up by doing the same examination with the patient now in the anatomical position. This not only reminds me what makes sense, but also gives the semi-astute chancer the opportunity to change the findings . . .

CYNICAL TIP 5: DRUGS DO EXACTLY WHAT THEY SAY ON THE TIN

Not all of them, of course. We're not talking drugs that give you energy, restore your vitality, smooth out your wrinkles and make you more attractive to the opposite sex (plus ensure you're better . . . equipped to deal with all that that entails . . .). Proper drugs. Drugs that you prescribe for people. I am immediately aware that these are exactly the sort of drugs that don't actually say what they do, on the tin – but you know what I mean.

Take anti-inflammatories ('Somebody! *Please* take anti- . . .'). They cut down inflammation in joints and make them feel *much* better. Of course, they're not the mainstay management of, say, rheumatoid arthritis 'cos we rheumatologists like to think we can hit the disease process earlier ('hit them where it doesn't hurt'), protecting joints from damage and that sort of thing

13 This refers to the patient. From the doctor's point of view, pretty much all examinations should be performed from a non-anatomical position . . . except maybe Romberg's test.

by using DMARDs (Disease-Modifying Anti-Rheumatic Drugs). We often compare these, both conventional (methotrexate, etc.) and 'biologic'[14] (anti-TNFs, etc.), using their ability to produce an 'ACR20' or 'ACR50' response – a 20% or 50% improvement respectively in a number of parameters such as joint pain, stiffness, number of swollen joints – that sort of stuff. Good drugs can get 50–60% of patients achieving an ACR20 response. That's very impressive. But why am I telling you all this? Well, here's a thing. Few people realise this ACR20 is pretty much the same response you almost always get when the patient first toddles off to the chemist and buys some ibuprofen. Of course, the DMARD responses are on top of this effect, but the fact remains that NSAIDs make a huge difference to the symptoms of inflammatory arthritis (as shown in satisfyingly sadistic fashion when you stop these drugs in a trial). Even miserably bad arthritis. Let's face it, they make *gout* better.

So what makes this a *cynical* tip?

Well, while *I* know the above, and now *you* know the above (assuming you believe me), the patient doesn't (there's that hook again). He/she thinks that proper arthritis won't be helped by anti-inflammatories. So if he/she hasn't much wrong with them, but wants to impress you with how bad their arthritis is, they'll say that anti-inflammatories are no help at all. Whereupon, in the absence of any convincing evidence to the contrary (such as a red knee the size of a football), you'll know they don't have inflammatory arthritis.

This doesn't necessarily mean they don't have pain, but that's another story.

PS Other drugs that do what they claim include analgesics. Painkillers kill pain. Particularly pain of organic cause. A headache which is initially helped by paracetamol is more suggestive of something proper going on, like a space-occupying lesion, than one where the tablets 'never touch it'.

PPS Beta-blockers slow the heart. If it's going at 95/min, you're not taking them (or you're very, very upset).

---

14 Patients are dead keen to get 'biologicals'. I blame the washing-powder ads of the 60s and 70s.

CYNICAL TIP 6: YOU CAN GET SIDE EFFECTS FROM ALL THE DRUGS SOME OF THE TIME . . .

Any drug can cause side effects. Otherwise, you can't take it seriously as a drug. This is something you occasionally have to remind alternative medicine enthusiasts – e.g. that if *Amelanchier lamarckii* root really does have active effects on the body and can knock Viagra into a cocked hat, then it will also have potential for side effects (actually a really weird burning sensation on your left elbow . . .) – but in general is accepted by everyone as a fact.

Some drugs will give you side effects all the time (like steroids). All drugs will give you side effects some of the time. But not all drugs will give you side effects all of the time. Not in any patient.

And the tip?

If your patient gets a side effect with every single drug that you try to treat their disease with . . . THEY DON'T WANT THEIR DISEASE TREATED.

Seems weird, but there are possible reasons.

They may be petrified of all drugs, and only ever agree to take one just to keep the doctor happy – but will then stop them at the flimsiest excuse. More perversely, it *might* be because they like having the disease. There are tales of patients omitting their anticonvulsant medication because they miss the 'buzz' a seizure gives them (ECT has, after all, been used to treat depression).

But most likely, and the reason that makes this tip 'cynical', is that they have nothing much wrong with them. Whilst it might suit them financially, socially or otherwise to 'fool' you into saying they've got a particular disease (or at least admitting to the possibility), they're not daft. And taking the chance of dangerous side effects from a powerful drug, just to keep up appearances (back to that burning elbow again) won't necessarily be Plan A.

Awareness of this tip might save you going through a list of more and more unusual drugs you know less and less about, trying to treat a quasi-existent disease. Of course, some patients do have side effects with a number of drugs, but, as with lucky (or, indeed, unlucky) gamblers, the odds and probabilities should eventually catch up with them. Anything else is suspicious, and you should keep a particular eye out for:

1 Side effects always beginning within a week or two of starting the drug.
2 Side effects being consistently subjective (e.g. itch – yes, rash – no).
3 Same side effect (occasionally bizarre) with very different drugs (e.g. urinary frequency with sulphasalazine, then methotrexate).
4 Very different side effects with lots of very different drugs (especially if with point 5).

5 Patient pointing out side effect is on the manufacturer's leaflet-thingy. Particularly:
   5a Side effects that are apparently a misunderstanding of the side effects in the leaflet-thingy (e.g. a patient whose eyes hurt her in the sunshine when she takes a drug with 'photosensitivity' on its card).
6 Patient having been worried about this particular side effect with this particular drug before starting it.

Of course, none of these *per se* says the side effect isn't genuine (to be fair, the side effects on the manufacturer's leaflet-thingy are there for a reason[15]), but just be aware of the possibility.

Note the therapeutic plan is *never* to continue the drug with the dubious side effect – that's not what this is about. It's about what to do next. Whether or not it should be urgently replaced by another potentially toxic drug which might genuinely make the patient ill before they have time to drum up a dubious side effect.

. . . or whether the patient needs a short break.

CYNICAL TIP 7: NO ONE GETS A PERFECT 10

I'm not sure if this tip counts.

I've never actually used it, you see. Not as such. It has kinda cropped up when patients have volunteered the information and I've gone '. . . aha! . . .' – though very quietly and thoughtfully so they see it as some sort of empathetic rejoinder (have been working on my looking-empathetic skills . . . one day I'll work on my empathy skills). However, I have not yet used it as a deliberate manoeuvre.

But my daughter – the one with the recently broken foot – has just told me that they asked her at the hospital how bad the pain was – on a scale of one to ten (I correctly guessed she was an eight, but that's another story of infallible clinical acumen). Presumably they're doing some sort of survey to see if fractured metacarpals rate higher on a cosmic scale than crushed naviculars, sprained deltoid ligaments, or toes which have been accidentally put through a combine harvester (a *nine*). I innocently pointed out '. . . and if you say it's a ten, they know you're *at it*.'

And only then realised . . . what a good tip!

---

15 Which, incidentally, is nothing to do with patients avoiding side effects and everything to do with the manufacturers avoiding liability.

Everybody who has any sense would always leave space for a worse pain.

Whenever a patient in the past has volunteered the concept that their pain is the worst pain in the world and on a scale of one to ten would be a ten . . . there has been very little wrong with them.

So next time you have the rheumatologically challenged patient at your clinic, ask them to categorise their pain as above.

If it's a 'ten', they're at it.

If it's an 'eleven', they're at it, and not funny.

CYNICAL TIP 8: DOCTORS ARE PEOPLE TOO . . .

We are often reminded (not necessarily unnecessarily) that touching a patient, e.g. to examine them, is essentially an invasion of their personal space/self/privacy/autonomy/whatever and is not to be taken lightly (though I find the common referral to such things as 'a privilege' is itself an unwarranted assault on the English language).

It is rare for this to happen in the opposite direction. But occasionally patients do touch your person . . . often as a friendly gesture, perhaps as a way of saying they appreciate your efforts in a more meaningful way than normal. The only time it tends to irritate (other than the genuine violent assault) is the rare use of the doctor's body to demonstrate where their (i.e. the patient's) pains are – despite the implicit presence of a perfectly good body of their own which they could just as easily have pointed to. Years of low-frequency experience of this myself, plus discussion with my colleagues, has produced the conclusion that not only is this behaviour bizarre, it is also rarely accompanied by organic disease.

So the tip is:

➤ If the patient pokes bits of *your* body to show you just where *their* pains are, they haven't got any.

➤ If they squeeze a bit of your body quite hard to show you just how sore their pains are (*did* happen!), call the cops (*didn't* . . . must learn to put my moaning where my mouth is).

CYNICAL TIP 9: PAIN DOESN'T MAKE YOU SIGH

Well, not usually.

When Batman clobbers one of the Penguin's goons with his Utility-Belt-Buckle (**POW!**) then what happens is that the goon goes **OUCH!** or **AAARGH!**, or maybe, if he's been smacked on the mouth, **GMMMMPH!** – but what they don't go is '*s-i-g-h-h-h-h-h-* . . .'

One might make the case that the above pains are all of the rather 'acute' variety (even in slo-mo) and we may expect the '*sigh* . . .' reaction to more chronic discomforts. But even then, it's a chronic reaction to a chronic discomfort, and the sudden intermittent frequent sighing of some patients attending the clinic every time they move, or sit up, or start a new phase of their story, just doesn't suggest to me that this is caused by episodes of pain (not that I'm sure I'd be convinced by **OUCH!** either – despite being the son of the only woman in history who would sneeze making the sound 'a-tish-oo!').[16]

CYNICAL TIP 10: IF THE STORY OF THE 'EMERGENCY' BEGINS FIVE YEARS AGO, THERE'S NOTHING WRONG WITH THE PATIENT

You will be familiar, or *will* be familiar, with the scenario.

Post-receiving ward round:

> And what brought you into hospital?[17]
> Well, six years ago I had a stroke . . .

Which prelude (sometimes prefaced by the particularly irritating 'to let you understand, Doctor . . .' q.v.) is almost invariably followed by a story which has as much chance of being another stroke, or anything related to a stroke, as Vera Lynn has of having another number one hit record (. . . OK . . . I was unlucky).

Of course there is the occasional occasion when such a preliminary is entirely appropriate, but in general the presentation of a long-past diagnosis as an opening gambit means that the patient is aware that their current story doesn't really sound anything like any recognised medical condition, so they

---

16   I drew the being-convinced line at spasms of 'hic-cough!'
17   Don't panic. Nobody really says 'an ambulance'.

feel obliged to justify their presence in a hospital, hoping to channel your thoughts towards some respectable diagnosis which otherwise would not have occurred to you.

To be honest, this sort of thing usually makes me doubt the diagnosis of stroke (or whatever) in the first place and prompts me into an entirely reprehensible effort to demonstrate, by minute interrogation and examination of the patient in front of me, that the doctors got it wrong anything up to 20 years ago ('you don't look pregnant to me!'). Similarly, a patient with a dubious chest pain who mentions that they are on dihydrocodeine or tramadol for their 'arthritis' will throw me into an enthusiastic examination of their entire locomotor system, satisfying myself that they have nary a whiff of arthropathy, and thus adding weight to my suspicion that their chest pain is itself entirely bogus. Later, when their troponin results return and they are being whisked off to coronary care, it's no real problem to hide the exercise-tolerance-test tracing as if it never happened . . .

CYNICAL TIP 11: DOGS LICK THEIR WOUNDS, NOT THEIR KNEECAPS[18]

When you bump your elbow, your other arm automatically goes over and rubs your elbow. If you bump another part of your arm, it rubs that. Burn your thumb and you'll find yourself putting your thumb in your mouth, or blowing on it, or running it under a handy tap. Your thumb, that is. Not, say, your pinkie – or your aforementioned elbow. The pain tells you which bit's been damaged, and you take steps to heal it, or soothe it, or protect it. That's what pain is paid for. It tells you where the problem is.

Except, of course, at football. If a football player gets nudged in some vague hip-to-hip contact, then he'll go down clutching his ankle (note the use of 'he' here as female football players would be too embarrassed). It's more impressive. It's the area that can get proper hurt from twists and things without being hit proper hard. It also looks much more elegantly purposeful (cf. Degas) to clutch your ankle than to clutch your hip.

(My apologies here to the distaff side for yet another extended football analogy. It's just that I've never seen anyone go down under an innocuous slide tackle in *Strictly Come Dancing* – though there was that woman who, to my mind, kept winning through to the next round purely on the basis

---

18 OK, they also lick other things, but that's not what this is about.

of her previous 'bravery' dancing on with a sprained ankle in Round 2. I'm convinced her limp changed sides in the later stages.)

Same with shins. If it's not a broken tibia, then it's just pain and it'll go away soon and only a big Jessie will roll around holding onto their shin in the interim – so you clutch your ankle. Deco did it for an entire UEFA cup final. But there is a danger of overdoing this 'simulation' as it's now known (more correctly, the 'simulation' is the going down for no apparent reason in the first place [actually there is an apparent reason, there just isn't a real one], but here we're concerned with 'afters'). Rivaldo's career never recovered from World Cup 2002 cameras capturing him clutching his face after a smartly kicked ball hit him reasonably gently in the midriff (*excruciatingly gently* in slo-mo). Cristiano Ronaldo (is there a theme here?) almost over-tried a nation's patience with his persistent inability to know not only where on his body he had been hit, but where on the field (usually vaguest around the penalty area) or indeed whether he had been hit at all.

So where is all this football chat taking us? Other than directly to the next chapter, girls?

Well, basically, if, during a clinical examination,[19] a patient winces with pain, they should know where the pain is. So next time you are examining, say, a hip by bending the knee and then rotating the hip and the patient winces or cries out – ask them *where was that sore?* If they go all uncertain and hesitant before vaguely pointing towards a kneecap – don't give them sympathy. Give them a yellow card, and ask if they're Portuguese . . .[20]

(Alternatively, *à la* Wayne Rooney, you could knee them in the gonads and garner an entire nation's support for your innocence if they so much as wink . . . sorry, wince . . .)[21]

---

19 Rats! Was trying to break record for consecutive commas.
20 It's OK for me to slag the Portuguese. My wife's half Portuguese and I love them all to bits.
21 Ooops. Whereas, with the English . . . er . . . some of my best friends are . . .

CYNICAL TIP 12: IF A PATIENT SLEEPS THROUGH YOUR POST-RECEIVING WARD ROUND, THERE'S NOTHING WRONG WITH THEM

It happens like this (including today!): you're going round the ward, seeing yesterday's admissions, and you notice one patient on the opposite side sleeping . . . perhaps snoring . . . *perhaps* snoring most obviously when you are with the patient opposite. When you eventually reach them, they will not respond to their name, will slowly awaken with increasingly less gentle jostling of their arm, will exhibit some degree of surprise/confusion at their surroundings and portray a drowsy affect throughout your taking of their story.

This patient shouldn't have anything wrong with them you need to worry about.

Think about it.

Think about being a patient (a useful exercise for various reasons). You've been brought into hospital as an *emergency*. You have worrying symptoms. The doctors are not sure what's wrong. But the Big Boss is coming round in the morning. He/she will know. He/she is the expert.[22] He/she's gonna put together all the facts and come up with a diagnosis and a plan. Your whole world revolves round what they'll think, what they'll say . . . so you eat your breakfast and have a nap . . . ? . . .

You shouldn't have to worry about this patient because they're telling you *they* don't have to worry about themself.

The only genuine alternative to be aware of is the occasional pathological indifference sometimes seen in a patient with a subarachnoid haemorrhage. They just don't seem to care about anything.

There is another suggested scenario that the patient is very ill indeed. But that's not 'asleep'. That's *coma*, or *unconsciousness*. You can probably tell the difference (that's between coma and asleep, not between coma and unconsciousness). However, if it is the case that when *you* go up to a patient who is in coma and *you* twiddle their arm, they tend to wake up and talk to *you* . . . then you don't need any tips from me . . .

(Author's note: the patient who prompted the above tip later discharged themself 'against medical advice'.)

---

22   . . . we are looking at this from the *patient's* point of view. They don't know any better.

CYNICAL TIP 13: '. . . SINCE WE'RE TALKING ABOUT VEGETABLES . . .'

Er . . . we weren't, actually.

Not usually.

Vegetables don't tend to crop up in my in-clinic conversations with patients who have rheumatoid arthritis. But they crop up fairly often in conversations with patients who quite clearly don't have rheumatoid arthritis. Mainly because they volunteer that they 'can't chop vegetables' or alternatively (or alternatively and *also*) that they 'can't peel potatoes'. So I'm asking them what time of day the pains are worst . . . evening? . . . morning? . . . afternoon?[23] . . . and I get the reply, *'. . . when I'm chopping vegetables . . . I can't peel potatoes'.*

Now.

The fact that patients with rheumatoid arthritis don't mention this spontaneously, whilst patients with apparently nothing wrong with their joints do bring it up, might easily lead a cynical person to think this might be connected to 'chopping vegetables' and 'peeling potatoes' being specifically mentioned in DLA, etc. literature as the sort of activities that failure-to-manage might justify receiving some sort of financial assistance.

I have, indeed, sought out a cynical person and they do, indeed, think that. They suggest *'anyone who spontaneously volunteers having problems chopping vegetables or peeling potatoes won't have problems chopping vegetables or peeling potatoes'* as a cynical tip.

It certainly qualifies in the cynical department, and does have one intriguing observation to back it up.

None of them *ever* says they are 'unable to *chop potatoes*'.

---

23   Never put the important one first.

CYNICAL TIP 14: BREATHLESSNESS DOESN'T MAKE YOU SIGH EITHER

The original plan was to have this tip immediately after Tip 9, but the vagaries of publication have forced me to move it here . . . in a way unfortunate as the EITHER – already a rather (Caledonian?) idiomatic use of this adjunctive – now makes no sense at all. Of course, since we are by now at Tip 14, readers will be getting used to that phenomenon in a multitude of guises.

There's a thing that some patients do, apparently to impress upon you that they are ill. It's usually when they are trying to impress you with their breathlessness, but can occur in other scenarios as a non-specific I-am-generally-ill manoeuvre. It's a sort of sighing . . . fatigued . . . wistful . . . way of speaking that's supposed to suggest real effort with breathing, but sounds more like someone who's been listening to too much Country after their wife/husband ran off with the milkman/parlourmaid (or indeed, milkman/milkman).

You'll know it when you see it.

It's not breathlessness.

CYNICAL TIP 15: 'TO LET YOU UNDERSTAND, DOCTOR . . .'

To let you understand, this is also a phrase that may be limited to certain parts of the country. To let you understand why I've included it, there were problems getting to the magical number of 101 tips (to let you understand, that's not because I'm lazy, but because 101 is actually quite a lot of tips when you're trying to keep them all fresh and bright and new) and whenever I came across an interesting concept whilst staggering through my post-receiving ward round (to let you understand, that's not because I'm drunk but because they're actually quite lengthy and fatiguing) I'd say 'I could use that as a tip' and note it down for later (to let you understand, it's not that I go on and on about my tip book during ward rounds – but if I didn't say it out loud, I'd do something that wouldn't help . . . which was . . . what was it again? . . . oh yes, forget about it).

To let you understand, 'to let you understand' isn't really designed to introduce some information which will help you understand. It is a supposed-to-be-helpful apologetic phrase which means that I-realise-all-this-doesn't-make-me-look-good-but-there-are-mitigating-circumstances-which-if-I-mention-them-might-help-you-view-my-position-in-a-slightly-more-favourable-light.

When patients use this as a prelude or adjunctive to their presenting complaint, it means they know their story is tripe, that it doesn't make any sense or require an ounce of thought of the analytical diagnostic variety, but if you'd only take into account this entirely unrelated factor (they had a stroke 53 years ago [Cynical Tip 10], their father had arthritis, their daughter got married last week, their chiropractor was reading about East–West Venezuelan pan-encephalitis, their wife has just gone into hospital, their wife has just run off with another man, their wife has just come back from running off with another man . . .) you'll see why their entirely unconvincing story should be taken seriously.

It is usually a sign of NoWWT.

CYNICAL TIP 16: *VOMITING* HAS ONE 'T', *FITTING* HAS TWO

The first part of this tip is every bit as straightforward as it looks. It's a simple spelling tip (though not that simple to say . . .). *Vomiting* has one 't'. Might not seem much, but it's very difficult to take a doctor's clerk-in seriously when he/she's misspelled the patient's primary symptom.

The second part, on the other hand, is more abstruse than you could possibly imagine. *Fitting* has two 't's. With only one, it would be *fiting* – which would clearly be pronounced as in 'fighting', very different from *fitting*. Which they are – fitting and fighting. Very different. Those patients who have violent seizures where they're thrashing about, hitting every nurse, doctor and porter who's trying to attend to them – are probably not having seizures. At the more subtle level of the standard pseudoseizure (a seizure-like episode not sparked by epileptogenic activity in the brain, but usually occurring in patients who also have genuine seizures and who themselves cannot always tell the difference), this differentiation may also be helpful. If you suspect a pseudoseizure, it may be worthwhile trying to gently prise open the patient's eyes.[24] Normally, during a genuine seizure, the eyes can be opened easily.

If they resist, holding them tight shut, they're *fiting*.

---

24 On review, that should probably be 'eyelids'. To avoid any nasty popping sounds.

CYNICAL TIP 17: ARTHRITIS DOESN'T CAUSE . . .

Any time you feel your cynical skills going a bit rusty – perhaps some unwanted empathy creeping into your psyche ('going soft') – vetting GP referral letters is a good way to get back on the cynical rails. Particularly rheumatology referrals. Just yesterday, perusing the 'aches and pains's and 'bitterly complaining of pain's (why do they never complain bitterly of aches?), one particular patient was 'beginning to drop things' – prompting me to think: *arthritis doesn't make you drop things*.

'Sorry?' said a passing-through respiratory physician. These creatures like to come by and annoy you, since there's usually so many of them that after working out next week's bronchoscopy rota they've got nothing much to do.

I realised I'd been thinking out loud, and made a mental note to avoid that in future.

'I would if I were you,' he said.

'*Arthritis doesn't cause you to drop things,*' I repeated by way of explanation, 'so this woman,' I pointed to the letter, '. . . probably doesn't have arthritis.'

He looked unconvinced. 'Except . . . maybe they do when . . .' he mimed stumbling forwards towards the ground '. . . and they have to . . .' his hand splayed open, dropping an invisible item to the floor '. . . to protect themselves.'

So I was obliged to point out:

Arthritis doesn't cause you to fall.

PS Since writing the above, the patient has turned up (see? NHS waiting lists aren't that long – less time than it takes to write a book). A perfectly nice woman who does have something wrong – but it isn't arthritis.

CYNICAL TIP 18: DISEASES REQUIRING EMERGENCY ADMISSION THAT DON'T CAUSE TACHYCARDIA

I love lists.

It's a boy thing.

Right down to top-five-films-with-exactly-ten-letters-in-title-beginning-with-the-letter-C.[25] (since you ask: *Casablanca* (1942), *Cry Freedom* (1987), *Cinderella* (1950), *Caravaggio* (1986) and *Carla's Song* (1996)[26] – not necessarily in that order [aye right![27]]). But this isn't about making a list. It's about *not* making a list – or making a non-list.

Complete heart block . . . myxoedema coma . . . er . . . complete heart block due to myxoedema coma . . . er . . . more complete heart block . . .

Fact is, there aren't many proper acute illnesses that don't cause tachycardia. Spookily enough, the main one is probably myocardial infarction. Everything else, LVF, asthma, pneumonia, DTs, septicaemia, rampant nymphomania . . . if it's bad enough to get you into hospital, then it'll cause tachycardia. And that's worth remembering when you're trying to assess how bad someone's asthma attack is – or whether they have DTs. If they have no tachy, they're (hopefully) not that unwell.[28]

And, of course, the corollary. If someone seems OK . . . not that unwell . . . not that breathless, but they have an entirely unexplained tachycardia (the classic is PTE) – don't blithely send them home.

---

25 Orson Welles must be kicking himself. Should have called him *Kan*.

26 Since you ask again: a) because Hayashi's *Ni ju-seiki Shonen Dokuhon* ('Circus Boys' [1989]) was not English language and b) because none of the *Carry-On* films had a short enough third word.

27 A Scottishism. There's a story of a European linguistics professor giving a lecture to a Glasgow audience (?!) pontificating that whilst in very many languages two negatives will make a positive, there wasn't a language on the planet so meretricious as to have two positives make a negative. To which a guy in the back shouts 'Aye-Right!'.

28 Before you rush to put things down to 'anxiety', however, don't forget *that* tends to cause tachycardia.

CYNICAL TIP 19: GP SURGERIES AREN'T THAT DANGEROUS

Simple maths (or *math*, as some colonial cousins would have it – presumably they think the big word is *mathematic*).

Percentage of life spent at GP surgery by average human being – 0.0328%.

Percentage of admitted patients whose breathlessness, pain, funny-feeling-all-over began in GP surgery – 6.56%.

So . . . either GP surgeries are really dangerous places, and make you have acute medical episodes (exactly 200 times as many as normal if you believe these figures I entirely made up), or otherwise ignorable episodes will land you in hospital if they occur in a surgery. No. It's *not* because sick people go to surgeries. Almost invariably you will find that the patient has attended the surgery with something else (usually for a 'routine check-up' or blood test) including a relative.

So . . . either **1**) GPs toss patients into hospital with stuff that otherwise wouldn't bother the patient one whit or **2**) patients lay on symptoms a bit thick in their GP's surgery and either **2a**) get their just desserts when tossed into hospital or **2b**) achieve their desired effect when tossed into hospital since they either **2bi**) enjoy winding up people like myself or **2bii**) simply want a rest in hospital because **2biiα**) their work is becoming too stressful or **2biiβ**) their wife is driving them up the wall because **2biiβⅠb**) . . .

And you can choose your most favoured option based on your current feelings or stance *vis-à-vis* GPs, patients, or indeed, wives.

CYNICAL TIP 20: NP DNAs HAVE NoWWT

I'll go through that in reverse.

That's **No**thing-**W**rong-**W**ith-**T**hem.

This has cropped up already, so I really should explain.

When I first coined this seminal phrase of Cynical Acumen (OK – 'coining' a phrase that's probably been in use since Hippocrates is perhaps an over-statement) I made the rookie mistake of using the acronym *NWWT* (maybe I coined that) – looking back later in horror at the published article, realising it would read so much better as *NoWWT*.[29]

(Maybe not. Many years ago my friend slagged off the secretary of our student society [don't ask] for desperately trying to write up his stuff half-an-hour before the AGM was due to begin, with the wistful 'A secretary's work is never done . . . until the last moment.' I spotted he'd missed out on a perfect chance for '. . . until the last *minute*.' He agreed – though oddly, the neat pun seems to take away from the effect of the original insult.)

Meanwhile:
➤ *Have* is third-person-plural-ongoing-present of the verb 'to have': *hold, possess, own, etc.*
➤ *DNAs* are 'Did Not Attends' – or non-attenders. Used as a verb with *au courant* (Google it!) grammatical laxity, 'this patient has DNAd' means they haven't turned up.
➤ *NPs* are 'New Patients' – as opposed to 'Returns' – new referrals to your clinic, requiring initial assessment using your specialist expertise.

Now you understand the terminology, the tip's veracity is self-evident. And if they phone up after missing their appointment, saying they *forgot*, asking for another one – you probably shouldn't bother as there's almost certainly NoWWT. Refer them back to their GP who can re-refer if there is any reason to think there's AWWT.

---

29 Indeed only then is it a proper pronounceable acronym and not just an initialism.

CYNICAL TIP 21: OPIATE WITHDRAWAL ISN'T TRAINSPOTTING

Another one of uncertain category.

It is perhaps encouraging that most junior doctors have never been heroin addicts, and have never gone through the trials and tribulations of opiate withdrawal.

The downside of this is that their knowledge of the scenario comes from two equally unreliable sources – the representation of 'Cold Turkey' in various films and TV programmes, and the patients themselves. Since drama is everything, most film directors will eschew the current medical thinking that opiate withdrawal is *less* toxic than alcohol withdrawal, in favour of a harrowing representation of agitated misery. Since getting their opiates is everything, most patients are quick to support this view. Junior doctors will thus find themselves under pressure to prescribe opiates for 'IV drug abusers'[30] within seconds of their admission to hospital and will have in their own minds a vision of abject misery for the patient if they don't act super-quickly.

A few observations:

0 Don't listen to the nurses (comes before 1 as it's a given).

1 There is no rush. Do not feel pressured to give anything.

2 Opiate withdrawal symptoms usually come on fairly gradually. Patients who say they are *'rattlin''* but are well, with no sweating or tachycardia, are unlikely to require immediate doses of opiate (and are unlikely to rattle).

3 If opiates are required, then small doses, e.g. 10–15 mL (mg) of methadone will be enough to keep the patient well in the short-term. Gradual increase, if required for complete resolution of symptoms, can be done 'at leisure'.

4 Re patients already established on methadone: methadone has a half-life of around 20 hours (officially 8–59 h). They will not develop major withdrawal symptoms within 36 hours of having had their dose of methadone. There is no hurry to institute any therapies – methadone itself or otherwise – within 24 hours of a patient's admission.

5 Patients who are already established on methadone are usually continued at their normal dose – *once this has been confirmed with GP, etc.* (again, there is time for this). Do not take the patient's word for dose as this can lead to overdosage.

---

30   In many places 'IV drug users' is now the accepted PC term. But not by me – since that slack terminology should logically result in our giving all post-op. patients some methadone to take home with them.

6 Dosage has been confirmed. All well and good. However. If you've ever actually seen anyone getting their methadone in a pharmacist's, you'll know that they're quite 'reasonably' given some degree of privacy – leading to the occasional practice of scoffing half the dose and keeping the rest to sell on the street (think about it; if you need 40 mL methadone, but can get your prescription built up to 80 mL – that's easy money). There is a worry, therefore, that if you do prescribe this patient 80 mL of methadone, that will double the dose they usually have every day and may induce life-threatening respiratory depression. My plan is often to split the first day's dose (given on the second day of admission) into two, i.e. in this scenario 40 mL bd – then 80 mL od the next day if there are no problems. This rarely meets with the patient's approval as the 80 mL bolus will be enough to give them 'a hit' but the 40 mL bd . . . won't.[31] My own feeling is that our job and duty is to keep them alive and well, rather than show them a good time, but I have to admit this stance is controversial.

7 If a patient in a single day takes their methadone at the chemist's, later uses heroin, later comes into hospital and you give them more methadone, later discharges themself and uses heroin again . . . they could easily get an overdose of opiates . . . partly due to those *prescribed by you* . . .

CYNICAL TIP 22: BEWARE THE STICK IN THE WRONG HAND

There are two things to know about walking sticks (assuming the plan is to help you walk rather than impress Princess Eugenie and her cousins as you stroll along the *Promenade des Anglais*).

One is that if you stand up straight with your arms at your side, the top of the walking stick should be level with your wrist (it'll also keep falling over, but try to cope).

Two is that, when using the stick to take the weight off a hip or knee joint (which is normally the plan), you use the stick in the ipsilateral hand to the *good* leg[32] (that's the same one, the same side as the good one, like if the left

---

31 Apparently that is why most patients get >50 mL per day. Doses smaller than this would be adequate to keep them well (indeed could gradually be reduced) but the prevailing wisdom among addiction specialists is to give a high enough dose to produce a hit in order to keep them on the programme. This is not necessarily relevant to the in-patient scenario.

32 Some physios insist the opposite is true for the knee, but surely that's tosh?

hip is bad, then you use the stick in the right hand . . . oh go look up 'ipsi-lateral' in *Chambers*.[33])

As a good doctor, you should walk your patient through this. Bad left leg. Stick in right hand. You walk with stick going down at same time as bad left leg . . . then good right leg on its own . . . then left (bad) leg plus stick . . . then good right leg on its own. You walk straight, evenly, smoothly. Then show them stick on wrong (bad) side which makes you 'hirple' up and down, putting stresses on other muscles and joints and giving you new pains elsewhere.

Now, if you want to help your joints, you use the stick in the correct hand. If you want to make it obvious you have a bad leg, such that it'll be the first thing that anybody notices about you, you should use your stick in the wrong hand. That's why the supersarcastic-anti-hero TV doctor House (who, contrary to a growing local belief, is NOT based on my first book *Cynical Acumen*) goes hirpling around like a half-eaten haggis instead of just walking a bit slower than everyone else. He knows better, but he wants it to be obvious he has a bad leg (be he the actor or the character).

So if your patient comes tottering in, using the walking stick in the wrong hand. Either they haven't been taught properly . . . or they want it to look obvious they have a 'bad leg' . . .

CYNICAL TIP 23: VENEPUNCTURE IS ONLY MEDIUM-SORE

We've all seen them. Patients who find venepuncture (even when not being done by an Occupational Health Nurse) really painful. I'm not talking about needle phobias or the like – that's different. I mean people who find the level of pain produced by having their blood taken, extremely severe. They wince. They groan. Sometimes, they will produce tears. Surprisingly often, they will be the same people who have earlier claimed to have 'a high pain threshold' (honest! keep an eye open for it).

Now. Fact is . . . venepuncture is only medium-sore.

So if you have a patient like this, you really must view their description of other pains, including their presenting complaint, with some caution. How bad is 'excruciating' pain in their knee, when having their blood taken makes them cry?

Aha, I hear you PC-ologists say, *but everyone feels pain differently . . . you don't know how much pain someone's in . . . you can't judge . . .*

---

33 No lawyers out there to get confused?

But that's my point. And I'm forced to judge. I have to judge how bad the pain is to help me diagnose what is causing it. I have to know what 'excruciating' means to this patient, and if venepuncture is worse than excruciating, then their excruciating pain is less likely to be a dissecting aortic aneurysm. (OK. We've moved on from the knee example. Keep up.)

But back to knees – I've seen more of them than dissecting aortic aneurysms. Whether it's because months of bad arthritis make you inured to pain, or for some other reason, the bottom line is this: I've yet to see a single patient-who-finds-venepuncture-agony who has anything much wrong with their joints.

CYNICAL TIP 24: 'I WOULDN'T MAKE THIS UP, OFFICER'

This one is really an 'anti-cynical' tip.

I've resorted to the cop–criminal analogy as the tip's real title is a bit unwieldy: *Subjective signs that are counter-intuitive **to the layman** should be taken seriously.*[34]

Last week I was examining a man who'd been admitted with low back pain radiating down into both thighs[35] (why, I hear you ask, was he admitted under the physicians? Well done! Take that attitude with you into the A&E and half my work is done here . . .).

I did my usual SLR (straight-leg-raising) followed by hip-rotation (with knee held bent) which is about my whack for examination in this area. Both these manoeuvres caused apparent severe acute pain anteriorly on left hip (somewhere near the anterior iliac spine . . . though I don't know where that is). The pain was on the left, no matter on which side I performed the manoeuvre – and I did the right side first.

Now.

Pain in this area is a bit dubious. From an arthritis point of view, I don't really expect pain there when I move the left leg around. I don't expect it *at all* when I move the right leg. But then, *neither would the patient*. Nor any other layman. If he was making up a pain, he wouldn't make it in his left leg when I moved the right. This is a real sign.

(By contrast, consider the above manoeuvre of bending the knees and rotating the hips. Hugely stresses the hips and brings on pain usually even

---

34 Cf. symptoms such as paraesthesia and weakness ending at the elbow. Counter-intuitive to *us*, and therefore shouldn't.

35 Bilateral is not usual for disc lesions, etc. Some people think it might suggest malignancy . . .

in mild OA. But patients with very little wrong with them [NoWWT] think it's stressing the knees and will complain of pain there [if you're really lucky, right in the patella[36]].)

This man's sign was real. Scans unfortunately showed metastases in a lumbar vertebra as well as possibly in the bone of the pelvis itself, causing his symptom complex.

CYNICAL TIP 25: QUICKIES

Anyone who says they have a 'high pain threshold' has a low pain threshold.

Anyone who is described as complaining 'bitterly' of pain is bitter, not pained.

Anyone who made up their last disease is more likely to be making up this one (but not necessarily . . . that whole 'wolf' thing . . .).

And my favourite . . . repeated from *Cynical Acumen* . . . (can't not):

> Any patient with chest pain who volunteers (before you have asked them) that the pain goes down the left arm, does not have cardiac ischaemia.

---

36 Though more often they'll 'point', with the palm of their hand, all around the knee.

Survival Tips

'Survival' has lots of connotations. At its most basic level, I might advise you not to argue with a patient's inebriated companions in Saturday night A&E, or not to keep walking in front of the X-ray machines (indeed . . . at the level of suggesting . . . don't become a radiologist).

But most of the time we'll be dealing with more mundane aspects: survival on the ward, survival of your street-cred, your personal space, your integrity, your career . . . your clothes. And just occasionally, the survival of your patient.

SURVIVAL TIP 1: DON'T ANSWER THE TELEPHONE

OK then – don't answer the telephone *if it's not for you.*

I was really pleased to see this tip win a competition in a students' magazine last year. All of that 'great minds think alike' stuff prevails. The first prize – a copy of *Cynical Acumen*[37] – is clearly going to a good home.

At first sight, the tip itself seems problematic. How can you tell that a phone call is not for you? But when you realise that it generally refers to a ward phone, it clearly oozes common sense. Why answer a phone whose caller will not be interested in your input? As a medical student, you will immediately be embroiled in things you can't deal with, and be forced to search apologetically for help despite the fact you have nothing to apologise

---

37 No, it wasn't. The second prize was actually two first editions of the original Leonardo da Vinci *Codex.*

for. Once a nurse has been found she'll tut-tut at your uselessness, further denting your fragile ego and cementing your place at the bottom of the food chain.

As a qualified doctor, the tip holds true – unless you are designated junior on that ward whereupon it just might be appropriate for you to pick up the receiver. Certainly as a doctor 'passing through' (seeing a consult, searching for case notes, appropriating Elastoplasts for your private practice . . .) picking up the phone at best gives you the job of *being the phone*. This machine has developed through years of genius design and improvements. It's got this bleepy noise built into it to attract the attention of somebody (i.e. a WARD NURSE) who can help the person at the other end of the line. That somebody's attention is no longer being attracted because the phone is no longer making the bleepy noise – which is your fault – so you now have to roam up and down the ward looking for a WARD NURSE, none of whom are in much of a mood to be found since otherwise they'd have answered the bleepy noise in the first place. At worst, the caller will ask specifically to 'speak to Nurse McTavish' and you're now designated gopher to find Nurse McTavish despite the fact you've no idea what he or she looks like and so have to ask every nurse you (eventually) find whether they're Nurse McTavish until finally one of them tells you she's not here 'cos it's her day off and why didn't you just look at the rota[38] – it's hanging beside the phone!

So, leave the phone alone. It looks rude. You'll feel embarrassed when somebody eventually comes to answer it (after stubbing out their fag in irritation). But it makes total sense.

PS For those of you who plan a career in surgery, ignore the bit in italics in the first line of this tip. Surgeons don't answer the phone even if it *is* for them – unless it's their stockbroker or stepmother.

---

38   Known to all nurses as the 'off-duty rota' rather than 'on-duty'. A unique
     approach. But it goes along with their concept of having 'five more sick days still
     to take this year . . .'

SURVIVAL TIP 2: CHECK THE GAS MASK

No. This isn't a left-over tip from WWI.

Every now and again we have to get away from all the bitter twistedness and twisted bitterness and bit-of-fun-Dougal that is cynical acumen, remember that we're doctors, and come up with a tip that is actually designed to save lives. So this survival tip is actually for the survival of the patient. Seems a bit over-worthy, but the fact that it slags off the guys in the A&E department does make me more comfortable with it.

First of all, lets go through that whole 'Chron-Brons (now classified as 'COPDs . . . er . . . some of them' to any of you either under the age of 30 or in the respiratory profession) become-dependent-on-their-hypoxic-drive' thingy. Two things will 'make' us breathe: a high CO_2, or a low oxygen.[39] In the sort of COPD that we used to call chronic bronchitis, people who consistently 'retain CO_2' would eventually make their receptors (or receptor-activation pathway, or whatever) inured to the effect of this, so their lungs stopped responding to a high CO_2. Back in the old days, we'd all spend many a winter's eve with a jug of rum punch pondering over why these 'blue bloaters' did that whilst other patients became 'pink puffers' and got on with just overbreathing all the time – until those clever respiratory chappies came up with the solution. Stop calling them blue bloaters and pink puffers and pretend they're all the same and have all got COPD.

Anyways, these formerly-known-as-blue-bloaters breathe only as a response to low oxygen in their blood. So if they're struggling, and you give them high-flow (high percentage) oxygen, their brain will tell them just to take the occasional whiff – just enough to keep their oxygen levels up. This does NOT make them become hypoxic. Their oxygen's fine . . . they keep it up. But what they're not doing is blowing off CO_2 . . . so their CO_2 level rises, and hypercapnia itself is dangerous. But, as we've pointed out, they'll ignore that. So they'll carry on like this, apparently OK, keeping their O_2 just above par until they suddenly go into a hypercapnic respiratory arrest crash call . . .

Now we get to the A&E guys.

THEY DO NOT BELIEVE ANY OF THAT.

Their tenet is that people die of hypoxia, and nobody ever died of too much oxygen. They treat everybody's respiratory distress as though they've been hit by a red motorcycle and have a flail segment, i.e. with high-flow

---

39 They do actually 'make' you breathe. That's why a drowned person has lungs full of water. They will eventually be forced to breathe in the water by their medulla oblongata or somesuch, even though its smarter brother the cerebral cortex knows this is pointless and will not help them in any way – like buying the wife a Valentine's card.

oxygen. So that's what they'll give your blue bloater (in my own A&E, they refused even to have controlled-oxygen-type masks till we snuck in one night and put some on their shelves). And it seems to work – for them. 'Cause the whole hypercapnia scenario takes hours to build up, by which time the patient is unsafely tucked up in a medical ward – where at three in the morning they have their surprise, unpredictable, who-would-have-thought respiratory arrest.

So whenever you get a COPD patient from A&E, you CHECK THE GAS MASK and check their blood gases to *see* if they are a CO_2 retainer. If they are, then you can't give them oxygen willy-nilly through a Hudson mask (or 'trauma-mask' as they're called, in a vain attempt to give somebody, some-where, some sort of hint!), which is almost certainly what they will have on. They need a Venturi-mask ('Venti-mask') or equivalent. And if you can't see the label, that's the one with the lots of holes at the bit where the tube meets the mask, to let lots of air mix in with the oxygen.

And you get the nurses to change the mask until somebody comes along that can spell CPAP.

Careless Doc costs lives . . .

SURVIVAL TIP 3: DON'T ASSUME A RADIOLOGICAL DIAGNOSIS IS CORRECT

Particularly of metastases.

We've all done it. Well, all of us above a certain age (the age at which you done it). The ultrasound report says 'the liver is full of metastases' and despite knowing that this is simply an opinion (and, in the case of an ultrasound, one person's take on the relevant significances of thirteen different varieties of blurry snowstorm), our mentals are set. This person has metastases. We know further confirmation is required, but if, for example, the patient pushes us for the results, we feel that it would be wrong to raise their hopes too much.[40] Or if their health takes a turn for the worse, we think twice about aggressive management.

But lesions seen on the various forms of imaging now available to us don't

---

40   Exacerbated by the modern fascination with telling the patient everything as soon as humanly possible. If we used the old-school approach of keeping them entirely in the dark until we know exactly what is going on, none of these problems would arise and everybody (except intra-self-appointed PC doctor-educators) would be happy (well, less unhappy).

always turn out to be the thing they most resemble.[41] A brain tumour on CT scan turns out to be an abscess. Bone secondaries from prostatic carcinoma turn out to be atypical mixed osteoporosis and osteomalacia. And nobody ever finds out what the liver metastases mentioned above actually are (yup . . . these are all real cases), but the patient remains well over the next few years while repeated scans show them gradually getting smaller (that's the lesions – even the profligate NHS doesn't scan patients to see if they're getting smaller).

So remember. Imaging results are just one piece in the diagnostic jigsaw. It's true we should be careful not to over-emphasise a single result from *any* modality – such as biochemistry or haematology – but I think radiology reports are the most over-regarded. Perhaps because they're 'expert' opinions (*see* Clinical Tip 2) that take away some of our own responsibility to interpret things. But they're not infallible. Take it on board, but don't over-present its importance to the patient, or relatives, or to your own diagnostic thinking processes until the histology comes in.

And even then . . .

SURVIVAL TIP 4: THE VEIN YOU CAN FEEL IS BIGGER THAN THE VEIN YOU CAN SEE

Clearly the most embarrassingly simple tip in the world. Everybody knows it. Everybody knows that everybody knows it . . . and there lies the rub (another good venepuncture tip). Nobody would actually tell anyone this – 'cos they'd assume they know it already. Yet, the recent penchant for nurses to take bloods at the clinic has allowed me to observe that they spend most of the time *looking* for a vein, and very little time *feeling*. And, sure enough, they often seem to opt for one of those narrow, marbly wisps of blue rather than the firm plump vein that's just screaming out to be attacked.[42] Just because it isn't bright blue, they ignore it. And these are people who are *trained* to take blood – no arbitrary osmotic learning methods for them. They're sent on courses. So chances are that nobody gets round to telling young whippersnapper doctors to **go for the vein you can feel, rather than the one you can see.**

Still seems a bit of a non-tip, though.

---

41 Otherwise we'd all assume the Americans went to the moon.
42 Reminiscent of my favourite ever tip for students – that the JVP is NOT blue – so don't go looking for a blue column of blood, just wobbling skin.

So I'll add a freebie.

When you smack the needle into the vein and the blood doesn't come back into the syringe/vacutainer/whatever, don't panic. Don't go poking it to the right (ouch!), then poking it to the left (ouch!), then delving in further (ouch!!!) or giving up altogether. Just draw the needle back towards you imperceptibly (almost) and six times out of ten the blood will come gushing out.

Again something anybody who's been taking blood for years takes for granted. No idea why it happens. I could speculate re valves and back walls and stuff, but why bother? Just worth letting everybody know how frustrating it is watching someone who doesn't know this – especially when they're taking *your* blood.

. . . Still too short. Another freebie. This one goes against the grain a bit since it is entirely for the benefit of the patient to cut down their discomfort and clearly not the sort of thing I like to be associated with. But since I get to be a patient myself sometimes and nobody else seems to tell you guys this, then *do not press down hard with the cotton wool before and during taking the needle out* (unless you plan a career as an Occupational Health Nurse . . . apparently). It's agony for the patient. And *so unnecessary*. Just learn to time it so that you take the needle out . . . then . . . instantaneously(?!) push down with the cotton wool. It's not that hard.

It's not supposed to be that hard.

That's why we use cotton wool.[43]

---

43 Which rather reminds me of the old joke:

What's 6ft by 3ft by 1ft and full of concrete?

I don't know.

A mattress.

. . . ?! . . . why full of concrete?

I just put that in to make it harder . . .

SURVIVAL TIP 5: (GERIATRICS) ALWAYS PUT YOUR HAND ON THE BED – OR SOFT FURNISHING – BEFORE SITTING ON IT

'Nuff said.

. . . or, apparently, not 'nuff said. It seems that the geriatricians are still bristling over the chapter on geriatrics in my previous book – *'Chapter 6. Geriatrics. Ask the patient how old they are . . . er . . . that's it . . .'* – sort of thing, and they'd like me to extend this tip (which is particularly aimed at domiciliary visits), by pointing out that the advice as it stands does land you with the occasional messed-up over-moist (or worse) hand and whilst this is easier to deal with than a wet trouser-bottom, it would be best to avoid the possibility entirely by adopting their more stringent rule for dommies . . . *don't touch anything!!!* . . .

CW

SURVIVAL TIP 6: MOST DANGEROUS CAUSES OF ABDOMINAL PAIN ARE SURGICAL

We all know that some weird (and not-so-weird) medical diseases can cause abdominal pain. Unfortunately, so do the surgeons.

And while we think that the odd case of diabetic ketoacidosis (or odder case of porphyria or lead poisoning or . . . er . . . that's it[44]) is just something to keep at the back of your mind, or dismiss with a few simple tests, the surgeons build a whole culture-belief-system around it. And this belief is that abdominal pain is due to one of these rarities until proven otherwise and should be looked after by physicians unless it needs to be operated on five minutes ago.

This suits the surgeons, who can keep their working-on-patients to a minimum, allowing more time to work on other things – like their swing.

This suits A&E staff, since they can bypass the difficulties of finding a surgeon in the middle of the day ('Oh! Right! I thought you said he was on his fourteenth *tea.'*) and slide all dubious abdominal pains quickly and smoothly to the medics.

This doesn't suit medics, of course, since we're as lazy as the rest of them – just less brazen about it.

And, I would argue, this doesn't suit the patients. The surgical argument

---

44 Sometimes it's really obvious I'm from a time when *Private Eye* was cool.

goes like this: *This might be appendicitis, torted ovarian cyst, ruptured diverticulum, intussuscepted Meckel's diverticulum – but it might be just a viral illness, or maybe a UTI – so the medics can look after it.* My argument goes like this: *Which of these are the dangerous ones? Which ones are we worried about?*

If I had either a heart attack or a virus – we weren't sure which – I'd want to be in CCU, not a short-stay ward. If I had either meningitis or an atypical toothache – we weren't sure which – I'd want to be in hospital, not at the dentist's. If I had found a suspicious briefcase tucked under the Prime Minister's car, I'd want it looked at by a bomb disposal expert, not a car mechanic – just in case it's *not* a bomb – nor by a company director who knows a lot about briefcases.[45]

So if I've got unexplained abdominal pain requiring admission to hospital, I want to be looked after by people who know what to look for if I have one of the possible *dangerous* things wrong with me. And that's the surgeons. 'Cos that's what they do (they gotta do something!). OK, it might just be something you ate, or a bit-of-wind, that a medic or your GP could look after. But if you're not convinced enough to send them straight back to aforementioned GP, then the person who knows the telltale signs for the *bad* diagnosis should take the case. So this is another survival tip in two ways. Any patient with unexplained abdominal pain needs assessing, repeatedly, by the people who know what to look for. If they've been 'landed' on a medical ward, keep getting the surgeons to see them.[46] If you're thinking of sending them home . . . again get the surgeons to see them. They won't like it, but hey! – they want you to look after the patient. This *is* you looking after the patient. And yourself.

---

45 And I've never quite understood the wife's plan NOT to pack an umbrella, just in case it *doesn't* rain.

46 Of course, none of this alters the fact that surgeons aren't the brightest sixpences in the toolbox and you do have to keep thinking about the case yourself.

SURVIVAL TIP 7: TAKE A BRIEFCASE TO ALL DOMMIES

Another tip from the geriatric stable.

To clarify, a 'dommy' is a 'domiciliary visit' – where a hospital consultant, usually a geriatrician, goes out to a patient's home at their GP's request to give expert diagnostic, therapeutic and 'services' advice. An often useful manoeuvre, preventing unnecessary hospital admissions, it was at one time the mainstay of the geriatrician's lot. Most would do 10–20 dommies per week. This was also quite lucrative, as the piecework payments for these visits were relatively tasty.

There is, however, a drawback.

The consultant is moving out of the 'comfort zone' that is the NHS hospital and into the real world that is . . . the real world. With all its inherent discomforts and dangers. A brave person might equate the gradual decrease in dommy referrals over the past two decades with the decrease in GPs themselves going out on home visits – leaving them feeling less need to 'get their own back'.

But that's not me.

Instead I'll settle for passing on a simple tip from a 'senior geriatric colleague' (love that phrase . . .) to anyone planning to visit a patient in their own home. 'Always carry a briefcase'.

No. I didn't believe it either:

> 'Why?'
>
> 'Well, not only is it convenient for carrying your stuff, it also helps fight off dogs.'
>
> 'Doesn't it attract drug-seeking muggers?'
>
> 'You don't use a doctor's bag. Just a briefcase – attaché-case sort of thing.'
>
> 'Doesn't that attract jewel thieves?'
>
> '. . . Prowling the high flats? . . . if you're that worried, get a brown one.'
>
> 'Doesn't that attract opprobrium from your peers?'
>
> '. . . again . . . prowling the high flats? . . . Look. This isn't about sartorial elegance. It's about defending yourself from rabid mutts that . . . prowl the high flats.'
>
> 'Wouldn't an umbrella be better?'
>
> 'No. You don't want to be seen actively hitting the dog. A briefcase gives you the right down-force to keep them at bay whilst not looking like you're actually attacking them[47] – as it happens it's also useful

---

47 Don't forget that when it comes to public sentiment, dogs come above doctors.

against those muggers you were all worried about, as muggers tend
to be on the short side . . . though since you mention it, it probably
is a good idea to jam a black umbrella into the angle of the outer
pocket of the briefcase.'
'To add to the down-force?'
'. . . [sigh] . . . in case it rains . . .'

IL

SURVIVAL TIP 8: DON'T STOP THE WARD TROLLEY RIGHT AT THE PATIENT'S BED

The title refers to Nightingale wards.[48] For those with bed bays, don't take the
trolley right into the bed bay.

Reasons? Lots of them – with something for everyone.

1 **The patient** . . . so it's not obvious to all their fellow patients, visiting
relatives or window cleaners that any clinical conversations before or after
the consultation are about *their* constipation, *their* alcohol problem, *their*
sexual difficulties . . .

2 **The junior doctor** . . . so it's not obvious to the patient that you've mislaid
their case notes, mislaid their results, or handed the wrong case notes to
the consultant.

3 **The middle-grade doctor** . . . so it's not obvious to the patient that you've been
studiously perusing the wrong person's notes before coming to see them.

4 **The consultant** . . . so it's not obvious to the patient that having initially
intended to see them, you've decided against it because a) you've realised
they're not your patient in the first place, b) the notes are missing, c)
the patient . . . just . . . looks like trouble . . . or d) you've had an oh-is-
it-that-time? moment when you remember a golfing appointment. This
reason is also to the patient's benefit as it avoids getting their hopes up
unnecessarily.

5 **The nurse** . . . so they won't be tempted to go tell the patient 'that's Doctor
Larkin here to see you', before turning to glimpse Doctor Larkin shuffling
off home to watch the football.

---

48 Genius innovation by young Florence – otherwise the Crimean wounded would
all have been nursed in posh individual side-rooms.

SURVIVAL TIP 9: CLEAR THE DECKS FOR A WARD ROUND

This isn't very PC – to the extent that I only partially follow the advice myself. But it really does improve the efficiency and effectiveness of a ward round if you get rid of all the extraneous characters hanging about like unwanted extras in a crowd scene from *Carmen*. This doesn't include physios, radiographers and nurses ministering to various patients (though in an ideal world . . .), but to people who could quite easily be somewhere else at this point in time, going about their business.

The accusations of non-PC-ness (while welcome) can be gainsaid by pointing out this is not a suggestion that biscuit sellers, newsagents, ward cleaners, etc. are in some way less important than doctors – but a suggestion that the four different practitioners could ply their trades at different times.

If you've ever tried to discern a tricky mitral stenosis over the sound of someone selling the 'EVE-N-ING . . . TIMES!!' (or indeed tried to sell an *Evening Times* over the sound of a Grundy-Mason Maxi-Floor-Cleaner Mark IV – 'beats as it sweeps as it screams') then you'll immediately see the sense of this.

Also unwelcome are the variously noisy shades of disc jockey – so all radios (and of course, TVs) should be switched off.[49]

Patient's relatives should also be politely asked to leave. Just because your mum's got a bad back doesn't mean you should be privy to the bowel problems of the patient in the next bed.[50] There's a bizarre presumption that the confidentiality circle extends to people who, whilst not actually having any medical/nursing/other responsibilities towards this or any other patient, have some legitimate reason for being in the vicinity. As if they are somehow blinded/deafened to the patient's personal details.[51] They aren't and it doesn't. That goes for WRVS helpers, hospital library facilitators, newsagents, cigarette girls and stray bullfighters from Seville.

All of the above leaves you free to actually take the patient's story and to actually examine them properly, listening for murmurs and split sounds

---

49 A manoeuvre likely to meet with universal applause from patients since they're only on to please the nurses.

50 Note the clever pretence that I'm talking about *other* patient's relatives.

51 For no reason at all I'm reminded of the nun in the bath who hears a knock on the door.
    Who is it?
    It's the blind man from the village.
    Oh . . . well . . . OK, in you come.
    Hi. Hey! Nice tits! Now, where do you want these blinds . . .?

(and infinitives) to your heart's content, interrupted only by the occasional beeping of ECG monitors . . . respiratory monitors . . . pulse oximeter alarms . . . infusion set alarms . . . (though if I had my way . . .).

SURVIVAL TIP 10: DON'T KNACKER YOUR BACK CHECKING FOR KNACKERED BACKS

Legs are quite heavy things. The percentage of body weight in the legs is about 40% (a little-known fact which was not at all known by me, so I broke my normal rules and looked it up on Wikipedia). Remember this next time you pick one up to perform the straight-leg-raising test, especially an obviously large-looking leg ('fat' would have saved space, but I'm trying to turn over a new leaf, gently) and be aware you can very easily put *your* back out whilst checking to see if the patient has put their back out. This is particularly galling when it occurs simultaneously with the realisation that the patient has NOT put their back out – and particularly particularly if the reason you knacker your back is that they do that pushing-their-leg-down-towards-the-bed thing (when you are trying to lift it up in the opposite direction) in an attempt to impress you with how sore their back is when it isn't sore at all, but boy oh boy[52] is yours now.

So pick up the patient's leg with a degree of caution, perhaps even letting them take some of the strain – and be alert to any sudden attacks of surprise gravity.

Other times when you should be careful not to let the patient damage you include:

➤ *Checking power grip in the hands* – always give them two fingers to crunch, as they can severely damage either one or three.

➤ *Examining a gouty joint in an extremity* – my colleague was kicked in the face last week whilst examining a podagra[53] in a slightly histrionic patient who liked to emphasise their pain with a bit of drama.

➤ *Examining anything in a slightly histrionic patient who likes to emphasise their pain with a bit of drama.*

➤ Taking blood from a patient with hemiballismus.[54]

---

52 No, I don't say 'boy oh boy' either, but the more genuine options were . . . ? . . .
53 Acute gouty attack at the base of the big toe. Nice old-fashioned term. Saves writing all of that out.
54 That's the *patient* – you're doing this deliberately.

SURVIVAL TIP 11: DON'T BE *TOO* APPROACHABLE

I guess this is really for budding consultants – but since anyone who buys a book as serious-minded as this one clearly has their eyes on the upper echelons of hospital medicine, I think it's worth including. Particularly since I first came across the concept back in the days of my 'residency' where two or three of us would share the responsibility for a big expansive ward (nowadays there would only be the one 'FY1'[55] for the ward, and he'll be leaving at half past ten to cover the coronary care unit – but at least he'll get away at half past eleven because he's been in *two days in a row* and he'll be going onto nights starting next Friday doing the late-middle-*fin de siècle* shift which leads into his annual leave slot in the run up to Christmas . . .)

Anyways . . . back then, if you were the resident who answered your page promptly and was willing to come round quite quickly to take bloods, or set up drips, or give IV drugs, or do an ECG (spot the odd one out[56]) then this fact would quickly be picked up by the nursing staff. Soon they wouldn't dream of calling up the other resident since that would waste valuable time and either delay the procedure or prevent it happening at all. So the diligent doctor got *much more work to do*, whilst I was in the mess playing snooker, trying to catch up on a *spent* youth (Hands up. Who all thought I was the other one?).[57]

Plus ça change. As a consultant, if you're more accessible than your colleagues – be they cardiologists, gastroenterologists, respiratory physicians – people will start to bypass them for any advice, referrals, basic monkey-passing. So you must adopt a certain degree of inflexibility, aloofness, diffidence . . . basically grumpiness. Don't go too far the other way. If there's three guys in your specialty, you don't want to be the one everybody slags off as being grumpy and lazy any more than you want to be the one who gets asked to do everything. There's always a Happy Medium.[58]

---

55 Sorry but I just can't stop thinking that's something the American Air Force sends out to kill people. Oh.
56 *Setting up drips*. It's the one juniors still get to do.
57 Come on . . . surely somebody!
58 Able to conjure up Spirits when required for effect, but not relentlessly plagued by them. For a fine (though depressing) portrayal of an Unhappy Medium, try Hilary Mantel's *Beyond Black*.

SURVIVAL TIP 12: 'HOW ARE ALL THE/MY/YOUR PATIENTS (DOING)?'

This is for juniors phoning a ward they are covering when they are *very* keen not to go there to do anything (cynical seniors may argue *'that's all the time'*, but let's try to keep this friendly). It is perhaps more geared to the good old days when a resident would be on call for non-receiving wards, and could sit watching TV all evening with a few like-minded buddies as long as the wards were quiet. Nowadays, of course, all your time on call is spent furiously working (*'so how come they're never in the ward'* – stop it you guys!) but you may be angling for a particular break to coincide with, say, your favourite TV programme.

The point is to use the title phraseology exactly as written (the *the/my/your* varies depending on the level of your connection with the ward, the optional *doing* depends on how abrupt your personal style makes the question sound without it). No 'any problems?' or 'is everybody OK?' options allowed. This isn't some PC, modern, 'think positive' approach thing. Much more pragmatic. Just look at the results:

> 'Any problems?'
> 'Well . . . Mr Smith has got his tummy ache again and Mr Jones . . .'

or

> 'Do you need me for anything?'
> 'Well . . . Mr Jones is needing his catheter changed, and Mr Brown has
> an awful . . .'

or

> 'Is everything OK?'
> 'Well . . . Mr Brown's wife is here and she was wondering if she and her
> sister-in-law[59] from Canada who used to work as a midwife could
> have a word with you to . . .'

as opposed to:

> 'How are all the patients?'
> 'Well...... '
> 'Excellent! Thank you.'

Whereupon you hang up and go back to *MasterChef*.

---

59 That's her brother's wife – *nothing* to do with the patient.

SURVIVAL TIP 13: A QUARTET OF PERCUSSION TIPS

1 Learn the whole Auenbrugger story (you know – the Austrian medical student who 'invented' percussion of the chest having watched his wine-merchant father using the technique to locate the level of anti-freeze in the barrels[60]) since there's a good 5–10 years' worth still left of ageing clinical examiners (like myself) who lap up that sort of thing.

2 Practise, practise, practise (also practise spelling this *verb* with an 's'). In particular when standing beside walls. Percussing proper stone walls as against plasterboard partition-type walls can give you major confidence that percussion actually works – as well as bringing sudden realisation what 'stony-dull' means.

3 When you feel a liver edge, percuss the top border of the liver to ensure the organ is indeed enlarged and not just 'pushed down' by, e.g. emphysema (superficial upper border normally at sixth rib).

4 Don't use wooden mallets with a glockenspiel.

SURVIVAL TIP 14: LEAVE TIME FOR THINGS OTHER THAN MEDICINE

Similar in outlook to the final tip in this section, here we supplement that advice in advance with actual genuine tips for the real world of things-other-than-medicine gleaned from years of experience of trying to think about medicine as little as possible.

➤ **Bridge**: Don't think of a pair of little old ladies as an easy mark – 5% of them are very good, and the other 95% almost all cheat.

➤ **Chess**: Always play in the strongest section of the tournament that your status/grading will allow. That way you don't spend an entire dreary week facing people who are all playing for a draw against you.

➤ **Cricket**: Learn to bowl. That way you don't spend a whole day of misery looking forward to what turns out to be 12 seconds of absolute misery (and you get to spend 12 overs of their innings not fielding).

➤ **Drink**: In a restaurant, always buy Rioja if you're drinking red (because of its quality-to-price ratio) and Burgundy – go for an area you don't recognise – if you're drinking white (because it's the only white worth

---

60 Reprehensibly gratuitous insult towards Austrian wine. And presumably anachronistic.

drinking without getting heartburn).[61] If, on the other hand, you're the sort of person who drinks beer or lager in a restaurant, please don't let anyone know you bought my book.

➤ **DVDs**: If it's a film with lots of good actors, but you've never heard of it, don't rent it.

➤ **Food**: Taste everything as you cook – no matter what those crazies in Infection Control might say.

➤ **Football**: Don't dive unless you play for the team the referee wants to win.[62]

➤ **Gardening**: Think what it'll look like in 10 years.

➤ **Music**: Only listen to music that has a tune in it somewhere.

➤ **Poker**: Bad players can still get good cards (like the absolute toffee I watched for ages persistently 'stealing blinds' with rubbish cards . . . until I finally got myself into a position to take advantage of this observation and hugely re-raise him . . . and his pocket Aces. Patience . . .).

➤ **Rugby**: Don't.

➤ **Scrabble**: When trying for a seven-letter word, think of endings and work your way back.

➤ **Self-promotion**: If having unposed group photo taken, point at something.

➤ **Sex**: Chat up the prettiest girls first – might as well find out if *they*'ve got a good personality. (The often-touted plan of 'snogging all the ugly girls 'cos they're so grateful and therefore . . .' is clearly reprehensible – though I've obviously considered it a concept worth encouraging amongst the female fraternity [sororororority . . . whatever].)

---

61 Skinflints who think ahead may consider marrying someone with family connections to a reasonable, but cheap, wine-producing country (e.g. Portugal, Chile) and can use that as an excuse for always buying their produce (particularly as presents) over the years.

62 Or are an established English internationalist hero playing in Premiership match . . . or paradoxically an established 'diver' whom referees find too embarrassing to pick up on yet again.

SURVIVAL TIP 15: DON'T GO ON TOO MANY COMMITTEES

Survival of your inner self, that is.

There's a brilliant short story by HG Wells – possibly my favourite back in teenage days when I had time to read short stories (nowadays I've only got time for novels[63]) – *The Pearl of Love*. As I remember, the young bride of a young Far-Eastern prince dies. In the following grief-stricken days, he has her entombed in a carved stone sarcophagus (I think I had to look that up). The sadness endures. He adds a 'chapel' (probably the wrong word) to the memory of his beloved. As years go by, and his abilities increase (did I mention he had an interest in architecture?), he adds more and more stunning designs to an ever-expanding mausoleum dedicated to his one lost love . . . until one day, surveying his achievement . . . surrounded by his builders and advisers . . . he is aware that something is wrong . . . it just doesn't look right. He points to the sarcophagus . . .

We all come into medicine for different reasons (I spotted it as the longest university course before having to work for a living) but most include somewhere deep down the wish to be a doctor. See and help people. (OK. That's enough. Let's not get all wussy.) But once you become a consultant, people start expecting you to do 'management' things. You get called to meetings about 'reorganising the service', setting up *Multidisciplinary Committees* to consider 'innovative redesign' and you feel you really must go. Outside your own specialty, they'll suck you into *Discharge Planning Groups* or *Hospital-at-Night Planning Committees* or *Resuscitation Committees* – maybe just one or two . . . but it does start to eat up your time. Then there are the groups which don't actually do stuff but make preparations for what you might do in the future if certain things happen – be they unpredictable (*Major Incident Planning Group*) or not (*Winter Planning Group* – buy lots of snowshoes while they're cheap). So you really should help with at least one of those . . . maybe by trimming back the Wednesday clinic. Meantime the *Hospital Subcommittees* and *Medical Subcommittees* (can't remember which one is the bigger – or what the actual 'committee' is) beckon. These collect doctors from around the city so they can put forward views on NHS structure and reorganisation that no one will listen to (I'm not saying they should listen – just don't waste people's time getting them to give opinions in the first place). Somebody has to go to them – and it's now your turn. If you cancel the Wednesday clinic all together, that would

---

63 Yes it does make sense. You can snatch the chance to read 10–15 pages of a novel and put it down again. Short stories must be read in one sitting so you need more time on your hands.

be OK – and then maybe you could do the CD-management role more properly. The SpR could cover the Friday clinic when necessary (he's very good and already does the ward round while you're at the *Audit Committee* meetings) . . . but now that the *Drugs and Therapeutics* guys would like you to head up the subcommittee that manages the formulary (though not the antibiotics' formulary which is obviously the remit of the *Antimicrobials' Subcommittee* – which you can liaise with and attend meetings of[64]) which could meet only on a Monday since your SIGN guideline commitments and *Managed Medical Networks* are pretty much using up all of Tuesdays . . .

. . . but the Monday clinic is the only one you've got left . . . and it wouldn't seem right morally or ethically (and you should know – you are the Chairman of the *Ethics' Committee*) . . . but it's the only time available so you're forced to point to the Monday afternoon clinic and say . . . the same as the prince said about the sarcophagus . . .

'*Take that thing away . . .*'

SURVIVAL TIP 16: DON'T RUSH TO ESTABLISH A 'DUTY OF CARE'

Hopefully, the spectre of 'medical negligence' will not often raise its blonde[65] head during your career. Or, if it does, you will be on the (arguably) less stressful side of 'preparing a report'. Either way, you will come to realise that a successful (for the prosecution) negligence case depends on proving three principles:[66]

1 A duty of care was established.

2 Negligence did occur.

3 The negligence was what led to the poor outcome ('causation').

The third aspect is often a fruitful source of defence. Even if it's clear you *should* have remembered to give the patient his antibiotic, if the exploding gas cooker in the hospital kitchen is what killed him, you will not be held

---

64 It's OK to end a bracketed sentence with a preposition. (That you can trust me with.)

65 Previously established as synonymous with 'ugly' (*Cynical Acumen*, p. 85). Blondes presumably appear agreeable because it's the only 'agreeable' adjective in English.

66 Note this is for legal cases. Being sued, etc. GMC cases, on the other hand, arguably come down to what they think *looks bad* and whether you need to be made an example of – the public image of doctors taking precedence over justice.

responsible (extreme example to simplify things – but if the patient's infection was so severe that the antibiotic could never have made any difference, that's when the principle can help you).

But the first can also be of some interest. Only if you establish the 'doctor–patient relationship' in the first place can you even think about being properly responsible for . . . your mistakes. This doesn't mean that the surgical ploy of never-actually-taking-over-the-care-of-a-patient-with-a-ruptured-diverticular-abscess-until-the-physicians-have-cured-their-osteoarthritis will avoid responsibility. You don't need to be the consultant-in-charge to be responsible for your actions *vis-à-vis* a patient. Once you see them in the doctor–patient situation, that's it. Even within the appointed management team, the idea that everything falls back on the consultant is another myth you should not fall for. If I'm back home on my night off having a bottle of Burgundy (coincidentally, as it happens . . . though otherwise not a good day), and my SHO hits a patient with an axe instead of giving them frusemide, then that's their mistake, not mine. Self-evident when you think about it.

So when are these opportunities to avoid the doctor–patient thingy (other than when any colleague asks you to see a manifestly tricky patient with 'trouble' written all over their Canadian daughter's forehead)? It's those good-Samaritan scenarios. Aeroplanes . . . road traffic accidents . . . theatre audiences . . . in all those 'is there a doctor in the house' situations, my advice is . . . *don't tell them you're a doctor.*

Everybody tells you that nobody in this situation will ever sue you – but why give them the chance? This doesn't mean you shouldn't help people in an emergency; just don't tell them you're a doctor. Say 'oh, I don't think you should move his neck' or whatever, and make sure everybody does the right thing (if you happen to know what that is. Onlookers who've done various life-saving-type courses might well have more knowledge about certain conditions than you do. However, once you're earmarked as a doctor, they might feel obliged to defer to your lesser knowledge[67] – highlighting one altruistic virtue of my approach). This might lessen your ability to persuade people to your views. 'Trust me, I'm a d- . . . deeply interested person in this sort of thing and read a book about it once' won't necessarily convince, but my plan would still be to keep the 'doctor' card up your sleeve unless absolutely necessary.

A sudden thought – and totally inappropriate one.

---

67 Cf. consultant passing cardiac arrest. My plan is always to go off and file my nails somewhere, and not get in people's way (assuming the people are there!).

You've just saved a gorgeous blonde's[68] life in a fancy restaurant by performing Heimlich's manoeuvre.[69] She is so grateful. Come and join me for drinks, handsome. She knows how people get together in *RomComs*, and let's face it you're far better looking than Tom Hanks. And you're her hero . . . so let's recap what you said to her exactly . . . are you also . . . her doctor?!

SURVIVAL TIP 17: YOU CAN'T 'USE' MURPHY'S LAW

Murphy's Law is a bit of an enigma.

It's difficult to define. I've heard the suggestion 'if there's anything that can go wrong, then it will' or 'always expect the worst-case scenario' – but I think there's a bit more to it. A touch of fatalism – or irony. Maybe just that there's nothing you can do about a bad outcome, or even that your efforts will turn out to cause the problem in the end.

So you can't 'use' Murphy's Law, or try to allow for it when making decisions. You know the sort of thing. The patient is on drug A and now develops a problem best treated by drug B – but 'once in a blue moon[70]' these drugs interact badly and '. . . knowing Murphy's Law that'll be what'll happen so we'd better use drug C . . .' (which is not as good as drug B but won't interact).

Bad thinking. You should follow the normal path, and not second-guess Murphy's Law. I could argue that this is because it isn't really a law, more a superstition, but I think its superficiality goes much deeper than that. First level of irony will ensure that any attempt to avert a poor outcome will produce a poor outcome. Second level ensures that if we allow for Murphy's Law, then this will be an occasion where the law will not prevail.

An everyday example will help. The usual one of toast *always* falling butter-side down. Never seemed that impressive – a 50:50 chance not going your way – but I suppose it's the accumulation of repeated instances that convinces (*see* Statistics Tip 2). There could be good scientific reasons for it – the buttered side being a bit heavier (denser) than the fluffy-toast side – but Murphy's Law as an explanation is more fun. Anyways, you're having toast and muffins with Olga Pulloffski The Beautiful Spy (told you it was everyday) and you know she's poisoned your toast, so you don't want to eat it, but you don't want her to know that you suspect.[71] So you 'accidentally'

68 I was only kiddin' earlier.
69 Only when necessary. First get them to cough, slap their back, hang them upside down (*mainly* with children) before trying Heimlich as last resort.
70 A necessary Lanarkshirism. All the hens there have got teeth.
71 Don't ask me. For some reason this is always the case (cf. *Prizzi's Honour*).

flick the toast off the table, and it lands on a pristine plate somebody's left on the floor . . . and it's butter-side up.

And *that's* Murphy's Law.

They'll be allergic to drug C.

SURVIVAL TIP 18: ALWAYS HAVE SOMEONE WITH YOU WHEN TALKING TO A RELATIVE

Relatives are tricky.

They've got all the 'moral high ground' of a patient, but without the dependency. Clearly, a patient's ability to cause you grief must be somewhat limited by their reliance on you for their well-being. To the relative, that is only a 'relative' truth. For all we know, they might not be that bothered about their granny's health, but that doesn't stop them from being in pole position to cause you misery. Even if they poisoned her in the first place – hoping to cash in on the Picasso over the fireplace to pay off their gambling debts – the whole politically correct world-view says that they can still give you a hard time, phoning up on their 'cellphone' demanding to know why the nurses aren't giving gran her digoxin tablets regularly.[72]

Even in jail you got to keep up appearances.[73]

Which is what most relatives are doing when they ask to speak to you. (Did I say *most*? Should I change that to *some*? . . . naah! . . .) It's not to do with concerns about their granny's, or mother's, or father's health. They know you're probably doing your best. But they've got to show their mother, or whoever, that they care about her. And they've got to show all the other relatives that they care about her. In worst-case scenarios they're trying to show their mother and everyone else that they care more than everyone else does (*see* Survival Tip 19).

So, speaking to relatives can be tricky. And you should always have someone there with you, for three good reasons. The first refers only to face-to-face confrontations, but the others I believe make a good enough case to justify having someone around even when you are speaking to them on the phone:

1 'Moral support' – it's universally accepted (though NOT by me) as a good thing for patients to have some moral support with them when seeing the doctor. When relatives are involved, *we* need it more than they do.

2 'Witness' – so that when you *deny* you insulted, were rude to, swore at, or

---

72 "Cos the bottle-full we gave her must be wearing off by now . . .'

73 I'm not sure the cellphone thing works. Ed.

otherwise abused the relative, you will have a witness that you are telling the truth.

3 'Conscience' – so that when you *deny* you insulted, were rude to, swore at, or otherwise abused the relative, you will *actually be* telling the truth. Having someone there will prevent you getting carried away (under any duress) and behaving inappropriately.

To be honest, I think all this might also hold true for seeing *patients*.

SURVIVAL TIP 19: DO NOT LOOK AFTER ANY PATIENT WHO OBVIOUSLY HAS TWO GROWN-UP DAUGHTERS

When it comes to competing to show mum who loves her the most by asking the most questions and giving the most suggestions and lodging the most complaints and making the most doctors' lives an absolute misery – two daughters take the most biscuits.

Or would that be three daughters?

My cardiology guru suggests this tip doesn't work; you can't actually refuse to look after a patient. But a lot of shuffling around goes on when you're sharing out wards, or beds within wards. If you can be the first one to spot the patient with the female issue currently residing in Manitoba,[74] you can stay ahead of the game.

If you're slow off the mark, make sure you invoke Survival Tip 18, and 20 if necessary.

PS This doesn't (necessarily) mean that *all* pairs of daughters will be nightmares. Note the 'obviously' in the title. The presence of two normal daughters will not usually come to your attention.

---

74 Have I mentioned in this tome that Canadian daughters are the worst?

SURVIVAL TIP 20: YOU HAVE NO OBLIGATION TO SPEAK TO RELATIVES

Not so much a tip as a statement of fact.

Use this fact sparingly, but have the knowledge of its existence at the back of your mind in all dealings with relatives. If you are being drawn into a confrontational relationship with a relative and your efforts to soften this are unsuccessful, you can simply break off relations. You can be held to account for being rude, abusive, etc. but not for not speaking to them at all. This may hopefully avoid the most popular complaint made by relatives[75] . . . about the doctor's 'attitude'. To my mind, this being a main complaint suggests that the doctor:

a) never did anything medically wrong;
b) never said anything that could be construed as inappropriate (otherwise it would be quoted);
c) wasn't liked by the relative.

. . . and that 'c' is the problem. Usually this is based on the 'arrogance' of the doctor – who presumably takes a stance that he/she knows more about medicine than the relative . . . reminding me of the time that Sir Alex Ferguson really hacked me off, acting as if he knew more about football management than I did . . .

. . . that pesky cardiology guru is at it again. Giving us that old canard about avoiding complaints by early communication with 'rellies'. This tip is simply a fact to keep in the back of your mind. It's a fall-back position if things are getting worse and worse despite your efforts (which you should indeed make). You don't have to speak to 'rellies', so don't let them force you to make matters worse by pretending that you do. They cannot complain THAT YOU DID NOT SPEAK TO THEM. In itself that is not a fault.

---

75 No. Not just about me. About everybody.

SURVIVAL TIP 21: DON'T JUST FOLLOW PROTOCOLS, UNDERSTAND THEM

This one's for the survival of the profession.

The medical world loves protocols.

Whether it's telling you how to manage a patient's diabetic ketoacidosis (*add potassium now!*), a pandemic (*wash hands now!*) or a student's misdemeanours (*wash hands now!*), the nanny-hierarchy is fascinated by the concept of pretty little boxes with prettier little arrows letting you know exactly what to do next.

I hate protocols.

I hate them for their presumption – that if I don't follow step-by-step the commands written by four guys who've never seen my patient, I'll make a complete mess of it.

I hate them for their limitations – you can't put all of the infinite variations of diseases, epidemics and people into your limited little boxes, so you have to lump things together, deal with generalities, miss bits out . . .

I hate them for their long-term effects (I predict) on the medical profession. As long as you can follow a protocol, you don't need to think for yourself. As long as you don't need to think for yourself, you don't need to know anything. Already, if you ask any juniors *why* you give the potassium in ketoacidosis most will have no idea – nor of why you convert from saline to dextrose when the glucose drops, instead of just stopping all therapies and going off to Starbucks. Soon they'll have no idea why you use antibiotics in the protocol for pneumonia (which will be diagnosed by noting three from five symptoms AND two from five signs OR an X-ray[76] report which mentions the word 'pneumonia').

Know the principles underlying the protocols. That way you can deal with the countless times the clinical scenario won't fit tidily into the pretty boxes.

---

76 No. Doesn't have to be a chest X-ray.

SURVIVAL TIP 22: DON'T SIGN ANYTHING UNLESS YOU KNOW IT'S TRUE

Out in the real world, this one's a given. You don't sign your name to anything unless you've thoroughly checked it. But we doctors seem to have forgotten that. A lot of stuff gets thrown at us to sign, and it's not really *our* signature that's wanted – just *a doctor's*. And we drift towards thinking of the signature as not actually ours, just a doctor's, which isn't so important.

But the opposite is the case. This is *your* signature, and the fact that you're a doctor is an *extra* importance. Things can happen because yours is a doctor's signature.

A recent ward round saw a Staff Nurse coming along and getting the SHO/FY2 ('needs an SHO's signature') to sign a form to admit a patient into the 'Chest Pain Unit' (before you ask, the CPU is a hypothetical state-of-being that we insert patients into so that the cardiology department can pretend it takes part in medical receiving and look useful). The SHO duly appended her scribble and handed the form back to Staff Nurse – who was rather taken aback when I snatched it gleefully from her hands and she was forced to witness the following conversation between myself and the SHO:

> OK . . . is Mr Bloggs now pain-free?
> Don't know . . . I think so.
> Is his chest X-ray normal?
> I don't know.
> Is the examination of his heart normal?
> Don't know.
> Is the examination of his chest normal?
> Don't kn . . .
> So . . . if you don't know any of these things, why have you signed a form saying that they're all true?
> . . . ?! [shrug of shoulders]

Now if there *is* some reason why this patient *shouldn't* have an ETT and something goes wrong . . .

Take your signature seriously. Including those times when you're paid pots of money for slapping it down – like cremation forms. The world isn't really giving you £50 for a mindless autograph. Read what is expected of you, and fulfil the conditions before signing it.

There's another side to this. Management knows doctors sign things at the drop of a hat – and they'll happily make use of that. So don't sign any contracts or other agreements with management without reading them thoroughly. They'll insert daft things like . . . their having copyright on any-thing you write on their computers (which is outrageous and would, for example, mean that you're lying when you tell the BMJ an article is yours to give) . . . bizarre new holiday rules . . . foisted 'uniforms'. In one hospital my 'contract' to use their X-ray software stated that if the system was in any way damaged by my usage, I would be *personally financially responsible* for the entire costs of fixing it. I didn't sign it.

People often say 'oh – they'd never actually enforce that clause', but if that's the case – as my three-year-old son once said[77] – 'why should that clause be there?'

SURVIVAL TIP 23: TRY TO SPEAK QUIETLY WHEN APPROPRIATE

I blame nurses.

No I *don't* always blame nurses. Sometimes I blame relatives, cardiologists, surgeons, management, the wife . . . sometimes I even blame abstract con-cepts, like Mother Nature, God's unbounded sense of irony, Problem-Based Learning (PBL), the wife . . .

I only never blame myself, but that's not my fault.

And the blame for this problem clearly lies on the shoulders of genera-tion upon generation of those self-styled Angels of Mercy. For years, they've shouted at patients (quite amicably . . . is that 'shouting with'?) as if they're at the other end of a long, dark[78] tunnel, moving on to shouting at each other whenever they're passing on information – be that a patient's bowel complaints, last night's TV, last night's encounter with Ward 14's Resident stallion, or last night's blunder when drug X was given to patient Y.[79]

Gradually, over the years, junior doctors have picked up the habit. Goodness knows how this 'gradually' happened, since they're different doc-tors every year (these days, every fortnight) but it has. Juniors attending the ward round tell you about the patient's symptoms AT THE TOP OF THEIR VOICES. Why? They mention the guy's an ALCOHOLIC . . . AT THE TOP OF

---

77 Back when he *was* three. My friend was showing off his new TV's remote (wow!) and teased 'don't press the green button – that makes the TV explode!' To which my three-year-old replied '. . . I don't see why that button should be there . . .'

78 No idea. Maybe sound travels poorly in the dark.

79 On the presumption it should really have gone to patient X – though the premise that patients should be treated with the drugs named after them is an unusual one.

THEIR VOICES. Why? They also tell you how things have GONE WRONG . . . AT THE TOP OF THEIR VOICES. Why? (Note this isn't an encouragement to cover up mistakes. There is a time and a place and a way of letting patients know when something has been done less than perfectly, but it isn't when you're halfway down the ward talking at another patient's bedside.)

Try to show a bit of decorum, professionalism, COMMON SENSE (sorry, didn't mean to shout).

SURVIVAL TIP 24: DON'T TELL RADIOLOGY WHAT TO DO

Compare the conversations:

1 We'd like an MRI of brain on Mrs Smith.
   What's it for?
   To exclude space-occupying lesion.
   Didn't we already do a CT scan on Mrs Smith[80] a few days ago and it
      was negative?
   But Dr Jones wants an MRI to make sure.
   CT scans pick up SOLs 95% of the time. It's rare for MRI to show
      anything different. We can't do an MRI on every negative CT . . .

2 Hi. We've got a 64-year-old lady here who's quite a problem. Had
   headaches the past few weeks. Started off in mornings, but they're
   getting worse and lasting longer. Paracetamol used to help, but not
   now. She had a CT scan four days ago which didn't show anything
   obvious, but she's still got the headache and some odd changes in her
   eye movements . . .

   This lady needs an MRI. If you send us a form I'll see if I can get you an
   urgent slot . . .

Don't start by asking people for fancy or unusual tests. Give them the story, let them know your difficulty and they'll try to help. They are doctors too. And they are people too. Often they will suggest the solution and it'll be exactly what you wanted in the first place – or better, since they know more about it than you do.

---

80 OK. Bad choice of name. Could be another Mrs Smith. But paradoxically by picking a random *common* name, I don't make it happen to sound like any real person.

And if you do want (e.g.) an MRI and they don't sound too keen (*see* Clinical Tip 1), stick at it. One trick is to ask very politely for the name of the person refusing the test. This can be enough to change their mind. It has changed mine in the past.

SURVIVAL TIP 25: NEVER WORK *TOO* HARD. YOU HAVE A FINITE TIME ON THIS PLANET

Honest.

Clinical Tips

Paradoxically, the clinical tips may be more controversial than the cynical. Once branded as 'cynical' the earlier 25 gems can be individually dismissed as 'what do you expect?', but clinical tips will be expected to ring a bell of virtuous truth. I feel it my duty to keep any such virtue in check, but adult doctors reading this tome might well expect to find 25 pieces of advice with which they are in perfect agreement.

Personally, I think that would be a shame.

CLINICAL TIP 1: LISTEN TO THE LITTLE MAN . . .

OK. This isn't my tip – but I'm going to use my most recent personal example to illustrate. From just last month, as seen via the conversation between the receiving consultant and a colleague:

> Remember the man who came in with his first-ever onset of atrial fibrillation?
> Guy in his forties?
> That's the one. And he also had that funny headache, or neck pain, on the right side.
> That had started after he'd been swimming?
> Right again. Crap swimmer – that's how he describes himself. Breast-stroke. Usually does 12 lengths, but this time he did 24 and got

> pains in his neck towards the end. Then it got worse afterwards, but had pretty much settled down by the time he came in.
>
> OK. I can see where this is going – 'Obviously caused by the swimming,' we all thought – so I suppose he turned out to be an MI?
>
> No. A cerebellar infarction . . . caused by a dissecting aneurysm in the
>
> . . .
>
> A what? That's a bit of a jump. How do you get from a-fib plus headache to there?
>
> I dunno.
>
> So how did you find out?
>
> I ordered a CT scan . . . that showed the cerebellar infarct and mass effect, so then we . . .
>
> Why . . . on . . . earth . . . did you do a CT scan?
>
> I dunno . . . the headache-neck thing . . . was . . . kinda . . . funny . . .

Maybe it's something you only 'learn' with experience, after seeing lots of typical and atypical versions of things. But maybe not. Maybe we're all born with varying degrees of awareness of when something's just not right – when the Little Man in the back of your mind says that there's something going on. You certainly can't teach it. But you can 'teach' one thing. When the Little Man does say something, don't ignore him.

PS There's another, more negative, version of the Little Man. He speaks when you're doing some procedure, or treating a patient with some drug and he says . . . *I think there might be a very good reason not to do this, but I can't think of what it is at the moment* . . . . Listen to him too. (This doesn't mean never do anything, just think twice when the Little Man speaks.)

> So, a lumbar puncture isn't anything like as fearsome as it sounds, Mr Smith. The fluid in your brain goes right down to the bottom of your spinal cord – below where the cord itself finishes, so there's a pouch of it down at the bottom where it's quite safe for me to put this needle here – see the size of it, not at all scary – into the middle of the pouch . . . and take out some of . . . did you say something about being on tablets? . . . 'warfarin' . . . well, in that case . . .

JA

CLINICAL TIP 2: DON'T BLINDLY FOLLOW EXPERT ADVICE

Four genuine conversations:

1 Consultant: Why did you change the vancomycin to metronidazole?
   Junior doc: 'Cos the bacteriologists said that's more usual for
      C. diff.

2 C: Why did you write her up for morphine?
   JD: 'Cos[81] the Pain Team told us to.

3 C: So why did you start iron tablets?
   JD: 'Cos the biochemistry report said he was iron deficient.

4 C: Why did you discharge this man home?
   JD: 'Cos the CPN said he wasn't a suicide risk.

Now. There are at least three good reasons why you shouldn't follow expert advice blindly.

a) IT MIGHT BE *WRONG*

Which can be very bad for the patient.
   As an illustration, we shall reveal the next lines in the conversations above.

1 C: But metronidazole was the antibiotic that 'caused' the C. *diff.* in the first place.

2 C: But she's got polymyalgia rheumatica. And we've just started steroids. By tomorrow she'll be jumping up and down and wanting to swim the channel.

3 C: But his results show a low iron AND a low Total Iron Binding Capacity – that's classic for failure of iron utilisation – his marrow's most likely stuffed full of iron but he's got that 'chronic disease' problem that won't be helped by giving him iron.

---

81   Note the junior docs use common-as-muck language with 'cos and stuff, whereas the consultant, having shrugged off his humble beginnings, uses his telephone voice throughout.

4 C: But he took a whole bottle of anti-freeze and locked himself in his car in the garage with a suicide note in his pocket and an exhaust pipe in his mouth and just happened to be found by a nosey neighbour at three in the morning . . .[82]

And the illustrated reasons that the experts get it wrong can be:
1 They don't know the whole story.
2 Their expertise doesn't actually apply to this case.
3 They're not actually experts, e.g. they're a *machine*.
4 They've . . . just got it wrong this time.

And every time, part of the reason is – this isn't their patient. It's yours. They're not necessarily looking at the whole picture, putting everything into perspective. They've no reason to. That's your job. And sometimes you've got to make a difficult call, and not just go with the expert's advice. It's not always that difficult, as it's often simply at the level of discussing things with a senior colleague (e.g. the consultant who *is* looking after the patient and who *is* responsible). Don't always assume that the guy you are working for knows less about everything than everyone else does.[83]

b) YOU DON'T LEARN ANYTHING

It's not wrong to follow expert advice, but wrong to follow it blindly – even if the advice is good. I get quite upset when the 'junior' (don't know why I feel I need the quotes, they generally are a tad younger than myself) hasn't asked the expert *why* they wish to change the management plan. As well as omitting to check whether the decision makes sense, it also means that, if the expert *is* showing expertise, neither the junior nor I will learn anything for next time.

c) YOU'LL UPSET YOUR BOSS

Obviously, if the advice is wrong as above, your boss will quite justifiably be upset. Even if the advice is reasonable, he/she/it will still be upset as their authority/autonomy/ego is being compromised, and you have to worry even if your boss is *unjustifiably* upset. There are three levels of such reasonable advice.

---

82 OK. True conversation 'stretched' for effect.
83 Generally I stand by every bit of advice I give in this book . . . but admit this isn't something I confidently tell my own team.

1 Clearly better than his previous plan. Then that's just tough. Your consultant can suck it up (though I wouldn't put it to him in quite those terms).
2 Simply another version of correct (a change of antibiotic to an equally effective favourite of microbiologist, or a move from diclofenac to ibuprofen). Then he has a bit of a case. Chat it over with him. Come to a sensible plan.
3 Totally counter to your boss's normal practice (Addiction Team suggest restarting methadone in patient recovering from five-week illness during which opiates were never required[84]). Then he has more than a case. Take him for a pint and join him in slagging off the perpetrators.

Think of the consultant as your wife (she-who-must-be-obeyed . . . it kinda works, and I've made him a guy to avoid misinterpretation). You're having the house decorated. She's picked a nice Pacific Blue for the living room. She gets back from work to find it's a Sahara Yellow. You say 'The decorator suggested it . . .'

See?

And that's even without you adding '. . . and he's an expert . . .'

So next time the consultant asks for an ultrasound result and you tell him that you didn't do the ultrasound because the surgeons saw the patient and said it wasn't needed and he says 'So-have-the-surgeons-taken-her-over-then?' . . . you'll know where he's coming from.

CLINICAL TIP 3: DON'T ASSUME EVERYONE ELSE IS BETTER THAN YOU (TIP 2 FOR ADULTS)

We all do it. We float an idea – a projected diagnosis in a difficult case or whatever – in front of a few colleagues. They pooh-pooh the idea and we discard it. Later we find we were right all along and feel annoyed with ourselves (hopefully not with our colleagues – there's no reason to be). As with Tip 2 for the juniors, it can also occur following advice from a single colleague, usually when a patient's case has strayed into his/her area of expertise. We will lay great store on what they say – and sometimes too much.

Why is this?

---

84 May not be cut-and-dried what is right here. My instinct is *not* to make the patient into an addict again when currently they are not. I might be wrong. The point is that since I am responsible for the patient, my views are (perhaps unfortunately) important.

I think it boils down to a desire to share responsibility – or even absolve ourselves entirely of one of the many responsibilities – 'monkeys' – we carry on our backs at any one time. You've got a lot of patients to worry about, and ceding the actual decision making (even virtually) for one of them lightens the load just a tad. The manoeuvre also seems to avoid the ever-present fear of making a mistake – though more often it's at the level of avoiding something that *looks* daft or unnecessary, like giving a patient empirical rifampicin or doing an it'll-be-normal LP. But it's always possible that the abrogating of responsibility *will be the mistake*.

The whole manoeuvre is very seductive, leading to quite bizarre acceptances of help. Witness self and radiologist recently discussing a freshly done CT scan:

> Radiologist: . . . and there are these round low-attenuation lesions in
>   the liver . . .
> Me: What do you think?
> R: Looks like metastases
> M: Could they be Strep. milleri abscesses?
> R: No . . . he'd be more sick if it was that . . .
> M: Ah . . . right . . . thanks . . .

No!!!

I've just accepted the clinical-situation advice from a radiologist! He isn't the one with the thirty years' experience of how anything can turn out to be anything, and he isn't the one actually looking after the patient. I wanted to know if the *radiological findings* could be abscesses and I've taken his physicianly opinion – based on a two-line note on a request card.

Of course we should always be taking advice and opinion. But we must remember that's all it is. Our colleagues, short or tall, friends or surgeons, are no more infallible than we are. We still have to do our own thinking, do our best to put everything together – and sometimes might just have to go out on a limb.

And now I realise – this isn't just Tip 2 for adults. There's a lot of Tip 1 in it too.

CLINICAL TIP 4: HOW TO TAKE A TRICKY BLOOD PRESSURE

I'm not sure about this one. But it did come from a cardiologist and I'd trust them with my life (though not my money, car, or wife – I'm sure there's an old song about it).

It might, for a start, be worryingly out-of-date. Nobody takes a BP with sphygmomanometer and stethoscope any more. Instead we put one of those bleepy-cuffy things on the arm and stand around idly whistling Country about our childhood sweetheart running off with a cardiologist until the bleepy-cuffy thing stops bleeping and we read off what purports to be the systolic and diastolic BPs. This despite the fact that none of us has the slightest idea of how it works. Indeed, often it doesn't – going through its whole bleepy-cuffy sequence before foundering onto an apologetic 'error' message. Yet when it does give us a pair of numbers – potentially random! – we accept them as gospel (unless the systolic is given as lower than the diastolic whereupon we just switch them around).

Anyways, do these gadgets make any sphygmo-BP tip out-of-date? I don't think so, since the very BPs with which the gadget struggles might well be the 'tricky' ones where you need this tip. You know the ones . . . low volume 'phut' sounds that you can't hear starting, never mind stopping (Korotkov5), never further-mind tell when they 'change imperceptibly' (honest – that's how I was taught) for Korotkov4.

And so to the tip. If you first elevate the patient's arm, then place the cuff around it and inflate, then let them rest their arm down, then do the whole stethoscope bit on the cubital fossa – the 'phuts' will be crystal clear! Dead easy to do K4 and K5. The cardio guys wax lyrical about draining the venous pool and stuff, but I'm not convinced they have the slightest idea how it works. But it does work!

Of course, all this draining-blood-from-the-area stuff must change peripheral resistance, etc. and will that make you get a false reading? Must go check. Where's my cuffy-bleepy thing? . . .

HMcA

CLINICAL TIP 5: THE PATIENT'S DIAGNOSIS ISN'T ALWAYS THE SAME AS LAST TIME

Another genuine conversation, this time from a post-receiving[85] ward round.

> C: And this next lady? . . .
> SHO: . . . is in with an exacerbation of asthma.
> C: What's the story?
> SHO: Well, it wasn't me that clerked her in, but apparently she was driving in her car when she had sudden-onset severe breathlessness and couldn't drive any more, and her husband had to drive her to A&E.
> C [RAISES EYEBROW]: And this is asthma, because? . . .
> SHO: . . . Well . . . she's got a history of asthma.
> C [RAISES EYEBROW WITH ADDED SARCASM]: Hmmm . . . I see from the notes she has three children. This isn't another pregnancy, then?[86]

Sometimes I think we shouldn't take the patient's past history at all. It maybe does more harm than good. Especially when we're happy to latch on to the first diagnosis that sounds vaguely like anything slightly resembling the problem the patient has come in with. And recent experience suggests this approach is becoming more and more common.

Of course, I blame PBL (Problem-Based Learning – it'll probably crop up again as I blame it for most things). This learning technique was introduced into our local medical school about 10 years ago. Groups of eight or so

---

85 That's what we call it. The day every punter-off-the-street belongs to you is 'receiving day'. Just up the road it's 'take', and Edinburgh has 'waiting day'. I presume different areas of England have their own vernacular . . . and all similarly preface the phrase with 'bloody' and 'sufface' it with 'again'?
86 Not genuine. *Esprit d'escalier* smart-alecism. Not that smart, either.

students[87] would come together one week and 'brainstorm'[88] a clinical scenario (No 1. A girl falls off her bike and the cut gets redder over the following days). They'd put together all they already knew, and work out what else they'd need to find out before next week's re-brainstorming and resolution of a series of set questions. During the week they'd hit the books (. . . hit the Net . . . hit the bar . . . whatever . . .) to achieve this.

The first year of this was understandably patchy. The group would run off at daft angles *('the bike could be made of lead . . . Charlie! – you go look up all you can on lead poisoning')* and the facilitator wasn't really supposed to 'help' unless it got too crazy *('. . . but if someone had been taken over by aliens, would they even be able to **ride** a bike? . . .')*, but it kinda worked, and at the end of term we'd have a colossal party and Mike would bring us all Big Mac Sundaes (just a check to make sure you're reading the footnotes).

But in the second year, the brainstorming all went outrageously smoothly. Sessions blocked for three hours would be over in 50 minutes, and the entire group could join Mike (repeating a year, but now shop-manager!) for early afternoon vegetarian fry-ups. Of course it transpired they had obtained the previous year's 'answers', and using this 'Prior-Based Learning' could now miss out all that faffing about with the history or examination and get to the diagnosis with slick efficiency.

Thus the PBL, having set out to teach the students to think-for-themselves rather than be spoon-fed, had achieved the exact opposite. Five years down the line, young doctors appeared who had been trained how to assess and diagnose a patient *when they already know what the diagnosis is*. This means you can cut out all that 'differential diagnosis' tosh and get on with managing whatever it was the last doctor said they had. Thus, a lady with a sudden onset of dyspnoea, which could be any one of a number of things which don't include asthma, will immediately be diagnosed as . . .

---

87 My group only had six: Mike had his weekly shift in McDonald's on Tuesday afternoons, and Fiona's educational advisor had discovered that I was facilitating and educationally advised her not to turn up.

88 Supposedly invented in the 1930s by an advertising exec-guy called Alex Faickley Osborn. But read this speech from the investigating judge in *La Mystère de la Chambre Jaune* (Gaston Leroux 1907): 'Since interrogation has given us nothing, we will abandon, for the moment, the old style of interrogation. I shall not have you brought in front of me one at a time. No. We will all remain here . . . We shall all be here with the same status . . . We shall chat! I have had you brought here to chat. We are at the scene of the crime, so what would we chat about other than the crime? Let us therefore talk about it! Talk about it! With abandon, with intelligence, with **stupidity**! Let us say anything and everything that comes into our heads. Let us talk without method, since method has not succeeded . . .'

And the moral is:

Diagnose and treat every case on its current merits – not past diagnoses (including misdiagnoses). That way you won't:

1 Dismiss as cracked ribs someone's bone metastases – that have been repeatedly bringing them up to casualty to be met with that same diagnosis for the last two months.
2 Treat a known porphyria-sufferer's ruptured appendix with IV fluids and morphine.
3 Help a young man with recurrent pneumothoraces fight off his pneumonia by jabbing a one-centimetre tube into his lungs ('. . . maybe it'll help the streptococci to escape . . .').

CLINICAL TIP 5a (FOR ADULTS ONLY): THE PATIENT'S *STORY* ISN'T ALWAYS THE SAME AS LAST TIME

Even if that was just 10 minutes ago.

If you are a consultant or registrar (or whatever they call it this week) coming to see the newly admitted patient after the junior, always take the patient's story *from the patient*. Don't go by the recorded history.

1 Patients genuinely change their story.
2 The junior may have used their finely-honed PBL skills to help them write down the story they wanted to hear in order to fit into their preconceived diagnosis. As designated adult, you have to be above this.

CLINICAL TIP 6: A LITTLE LEARNING IS A DANGEROUS THING

There should be a delineated 'figure of speech' for things that are examples of their own meaning. Like a superfluous tautology (not the greatest specimen, but I'll think of a better one before the book is published).[89]

People usually say 'a little *knowledge* is a dangerous thing' – clearly dangerous. If you're trying to play one-upmanship with someone it's unfortunate that you've just misquoted your own quote (from Alexander Pope) and lost face in demonstrating what indeed happens when you don't quite have the requisite degree of learning, or indeed knowledge.

---

89 . . . misspeling . . . 'euphemism' . . . tmbloodyesis . . . astronomical hyperbole . . . bathos . . . maybe not.

Sorry. Where was I? Oh yeah.

There are some nice smart-alec diagnoses available to us in medicine. And it's always nice to think 'outside the box' for that extra second and come up with the brilliant diagnostic coup.

A 15-year-old girl comes in with abdominal pain, and you save her from the surgeon's knife by diagnosing ketoacidosis-in-a-new-onset-diabetic just in the nick of time. Just remember to make sure she doesn't also have an acute appendicitis (or equivalent) that tipped her into diabetic decompensation in the first place.

Don't assume 'cos it's the smartest diagnosis it's the right one. Or even the only one. Always think twice when you find you've just said things like:

> . . . you can get that with her SLE so that'll be it . . .
> . . . drug interactions are generally overrated . . .
> . . . DVTs below the knee don't usually cause PTEs . . .
> . . . actually you can get anterior T-wave inversion with simple oesophageal pain . . .
> . . . I read last week in *101 Top Tips in Medicine* that . . .

CLINICAL TIP 7: THE HINNIEGRAM

This tip comes from an endocrinologist, but I decided to include it just the same.

It's all to do with that whole respiratory alkalosis/metabolic acidosis/respiratory acidosis/whatever-the-other-one-is thing. And what's good about it is, it reminds us how simple it all is.

I always get twitchy when juniors start quoting 'bicarbonate' at me when telling me about somebody's acidosis or alkalosis. Makes me feel inferior, as I never know what way it should go. But this tip encouraged me that that may be because I don't need to. I don't care which way the bicarbonate goes. It's weird watching people muck about with bicarbonate and CO_2 results and stuff to tell whether a patient is acidotic or alkalotic in the first place – 'cos that's down to one thing, the hydrogen-ion concentration: 40 nmol/L is the normal.[90] Range 35–45. More than 45 – acidotic. Less than 35 – alkalotic.

But which acidosis? Well, just remember that your body's tendency is always to get acidotic (for you science geeks, it's a bit like entropy . . . though for you knowledgeable science geeks, it probably isn't). All that breathing and kidney effort is an attempt (an impressively designed one) to keep acidosis at bay. So if you stop breathing, you get acidotic. And since breathing is 'blowing off CO_2', stopping breathing puts up your CO_2. So it's increased CO_2 that's associated with a **respiratory acidosis**. If you're acidotic for metabolic reasons like ketoacidosis (**metabolic acidosis**), you'll try to breathe pots and pots extra to try to bring your acid down, blow off lots of CO_2 and have a low CO_2.

Conversely, if you are alkalotic for some perverse metabolic reason (usually losing acid, such as vomiting rings round yourself[91] – **metabolic alkalosis**), your lungs aren't stupid enough to keep blowing off CO_2 and making it worse, and will quiet down a bit . . . so your CO_2 will go up. Whereas if you hyper-breathe for no good reason at all (or because some drug or brain incident makes you) blowing off the CO_2 will make you alkalotic with low CO_2 (**respiratory alkalosis**).

Dead simple.

And since I don't like tips taking the place of understanding, I've put down all of the above before getting to the simple tip for getting it right *even if you know nothing* (though its actual usefulness to you in orthopaedics is doubtful).

➤ Step 1: Do the blood gases.
➤ Step 2: The hydrogen-ion concentration or pH tells you if it's acidosis or alkalosis. Nothing else does.
➤ Step 3: Look along the correct row (there's only two!) of the Hinniegram for your result of CO_2 concentration, up or down (there's only two!) and it gives you the answer.

---

90 pH 7.4. Range 7.35–7.45. Asking juniors about pH is great fun. Remember **p** is the 'negative log, base 10' which instantly means nothing. But if I say the **p** of 10^{-9} is 9, the **p** of 10^{-8} is 8, you soon see how 1 nmol/L hydrogen (10^{-9} mol/L) is pH 9, 10 nmol/L hydrogen is pH 8, 100 nmol/L hydrogen is pH 7 – 40 nmol/L lies between those two (OK you have to look up log tables) at pH 7.4. But you can see how pH 7 and hydrogen-ion concentration of 100 nmol/L ring the same alarm bells. Just remember it's 'negative' log – so the lower the pH, the more acidotic it is.
91 Lanarkshire vernacular. Not sure of derivation, but always makes me think of being on slightly-too-fast merry-go-round in the swing park.

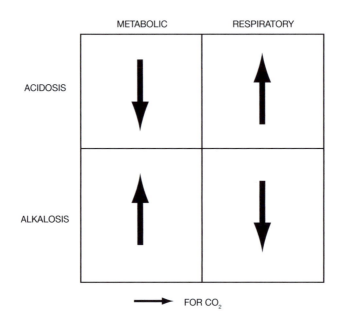

METABOLIC   RESPIRATORY

ACIDOSIS

ALKALOSIS

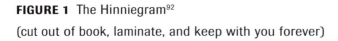 FOR CO_2

FIGURE 1 The Hinniegram[92]

(cut out of book, laminate, and keep with you forever)

---

92 The designer insisted on its retaining this name. Less shame than a shameless person.

If you lose the laminated card – and inexplicably don't wish to buy another copy of the book – then make your own. Simply remember that dead people, e.g. cardiac arrests, get acidotic (that's why you give them bicarbonate), and dead people don't breathe. So the acidosis plus $\uparrow CO_2$ is the respiratory acid-osis.[93] Put the $\uparrow$ into the appropriate box, and the rest fall into place.

Note we have not mentioned 'compensated metabolic acidosis', etc. Doesn't make it tricky at all. Just remember that your body doesn't compensate past the level of normal (why would it?) and use the absolute norms of 40 nmol/L and pH 7.4 instead of the ranges. If the CO_2 is all upset, but the acid–base balance is within the normal range, then just describe as before but vs. the absolute norm, and add the word 'compensated', e.g. H^+ 43, $CO_2\downarrow$ = *compensated* metabolic acidosis.[94]

JH

CLINICAL TIP 8: WHEN IS BREATHLESSNESS NOT DYSPNOEA . . . ?

First step is to be aware of the phenomenon.

A patient may – usually as part of a mixture of symptoms – complain of 'breathlessness' after walking, say, 50 yards. He'll often have some chest problems, perhaps heart troubles, but examination and tests such as arterial blood gases don't really suggest these are severe enough.

Just as your cynical colleague (don't you just hate them?) approaches the conclusion that he's making it up – or simply exaggerating – you remember *when is breathlessness not dyspnoea? . . . when it's* **fatigue**.

Lots of people, particularly those with some underlying chest disease, on finding themselves '*peck'd oot*'[95] after walking some distance will immediately interpret this as breathlessness when it may be fatigue. And even when you spot this possibility and ask them to clarify between the two – they still don't know which it is.

Second step is to know this question:

---

93 OK. Dead people's kidneys don't work either. This bit isn't explanation, it's mnemonic, and a platoon sergeant doesn't confirm his trooper has copped it by checking if his kidneys are still working. (Cf. *King Lear*: V iii 262; 'Lend me a creatinine analyser . . .')

94 Friendly cardiologist reviewer says 'so what about combined metabolic/respiratory acidosis?' It's OK. I'll replace him for next time.

95 A fine Scots' phrase which does for both symptoms.

> When you get this . . . thing . . . after walking 50 yards, does it feel as if you've actually walked a couple of miles . . . or as if you've actually run the 50 yards?

The second is dyspnoea, the first is fatigue.

And now you know it's fatigue, that's the easiest thing in the world to investigate and diagnose . . .

CLINICAL TIP 9: CALCULATING THE CARDIAC AXIS FROM AN ECG

First off, forget all that 'look for the lead with a QRS complex that looks like . . . a QRS complex, and as long as the other leads don't have any . . .' gunk.

The 'axis' of the heart is simple mathematics (once you remember how ECGs work), and you need look at only two leads (Standard Lead I and aVF).

Standard Lead I is the 'view' from the left-arm-lead towards the right-arm-lead, i.e. of 'electricity' moving across the heart from right to left. The size of the dominant upstroke (don't bother what letter it might be called) thus gives an indication of the 'leftness' of the cardiac axis – since electrical current going *towards* a lead conventionally gives an upstroke. If the *upstroke* is NOT dominant, but a downstroke is (still don't try to give it a letter as this is when it would get tricky, certainly for me), then there is a 'negative leftness' (less correctly, rightness).

aVF is the 'view' from a foot-lead towards a potential-difference-neutral point constructed by adding the potential differences of the other three 'tri-angulated' leads.[96] The dominant upstroke in this QRS complex thus gives an indication of the 'downness' of the cardiac axis.

We now have two different views (at right angles to each other) of the heart's electrical activity, and can give a precise description of the cardiac axis using the positiveness of these two for its leftness and downness. Thus if the R-wave in I is six boxes and the R-wave in aVF is six boxes, the cardiac axis is 45° below the left horizontal. It won't always be as simple as that. Strictly speaking, you should use the size of the dominant wave minus the non-dominant – that's how the transitional complex counts as a zero – and the angles aren't usually quite so obvious. But if you draw it out as a proper vector diagram, it always falls into place like Figures 2a and b.

And after a few goes, you don't even need to draw the pictures.

It's a breeze.

---

96 Yep. Means nothing to me either. But I did write it, so it must be true.

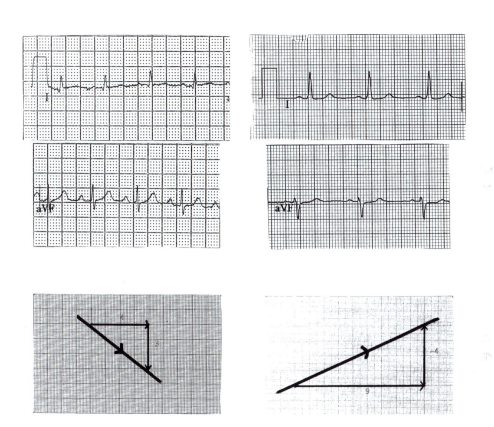

FIGURES 2A AND 2B Calculating the cardiac axis

Leads I and aVf from two ECGs showing vector calculation of the cardiac axis: 2a shows use of dominant minus non-dominant in aVf (6–3 = 3); 2b demonstrates 'negative downness' in aVf.

CLINICAL TIP 10: DON'T EVEN LOOK AT THE PERCENTAGE SATURATION

Remember that stuff they told you at medical school about 'iron studies'? With iron deficiency, the serum iron goes down, but the Total Iron Binding Capacity (TIBC) goes *up* – and the same applies if the 'transferrin' is the preferred accompaniment in your lab. On the other hand, if the TIBC stays normal, and especially if it goes down, then this is 'failure of iron utilisation' as in 'anaemia of chronic disease'. The patient is *not* iron deficient. Suck out some bone marrow and it'll be stuffed full of iron (nice image – and reminiscent to us elderly chaps of adverts for dog food).

Well it was all *true* – though even biochemists seem to forget every now and again, and label blatant chronic disease changes as 'iron deficiency'.

And another thing to realise is that the 'chronic disease' doesn't need to be that chronic. Just inflammatory.

Take these sets of serum results:

	IRON (N10–30)	TRANSFERRIN (N2–4)	% SATURATION
4.6.08	3	2.0	7
30.6.08	13	2.5	23

I showed these to a number of colleagues (who should have known better[97]) and asked them to *explain*. To a man, (OK 'to a person' – but it sounds odd) they all said that the patient had been given iron! But the early result clearly shows failure of iron utilisation – not iron deficiency. The mistake was to even *look at* the % saturation. Once the serum iron goes down really low, the % saturation will always be low. If your serum iron is 1, 2 or 3 or somesuch, your TIBC or transferrin just can't go down far enough to produce anything other than a mathematically low iron saturation. And the actual *explanation* of the results is, of course, that they've had their inflammatory disease treated – in this case, acute sarcoid treated by moderate dose prednisolone.

These are real results.

I'll say it again.

The stuff they told you at medical school was actually true (don't argue – it does happen).

Don't ask me why the iron studies do this – go read a proper book.

Just remember that the iron has to go down AND the binding capacity has to go up and only then you can make a diagnosis of iron deficiency . . . except . . .

---

97 a) about iron study results; b) about answering any daft questions asked by me.

CLINICAL TIP 11: IRON DEFICIENCY ISN'T A DIAGNOSIS

It's surprising the number of times patients will tell you that they have been started on iron by their GP, for tiredness, unmasking four potential levels of inappropriateness as:

➤ Case 1: Sometimes iron tablets have indeed been started for 'tiredness' without any FBC check to see if they are actually anaemic.

➤ Case 2: Sometimes the FBC will have confirmed anaemia, but there's been no check to see if it is iron deficiency (and lack of microcytosis may suggest it isn't).

➤ Case 3: Sometimes the iron studies will have been done and shown 'anaemia of chronic disease' – mistakenly treated with iron (*see* Tip 10).

➤ Case 4: Sometimes FBC does show anaemia, MCV is low, iron studies show reserves are low – so they are indeed iron deficient.

Only in Case 4 does iron therapy make any sense at all, but even here it has its dangers. *Iron deficiency is not a diagnosis.* It's a state. You have to find out the underlying reason for that state. It's like having a car which keeps running out of petrol after driving it for 10 miles. Yeah, the short-term 'diagnosis' is out-of-petrol, but you wouldn't 'manage' this simply by filling up the tank every 10 miles – you'd want to know *why* it was running out of petrol so fast.

In the same way, you can't just give the patient iron tablets to keep up with whatever the problem is. You have to take a history, examine them, and perhaps arrange investigations. There are lots of benign explanations – vegetarianism (but don't assume every patient of Asian ethnicity is vegetarian), heavy menses, etc. – but unexplained iron deficiency can also be the first sign of sinister diseases including bowel cancer. There's no room here to go into all the factors (age, bowel habit, other explanations) that tell you whether someone needs endoscopy and colonoscopy[98] ('topping and tailing' as your friendly gastroenterologist calls it) – I just want you to be aware that 'iron deficiency' doesn't mean *treat with iron and forget it.*

PS Please don't read this tip without reading the previous. Almost better to read neither. Patients misdiagnosed as iron deficient who have failure of iron utilisation usually come to no harm (though oral iron is not without side effects). Making both bloopers (misdiagnosing iron deficiency, then failing to investigate iron deficiency properly) would at least mean that your patients with chronic leg ulcers or renal failure don't all get bendy tubes with cameras, stuck up and down their various orifices. Two wrongs can make a serendipitous right after all.

---

98 Technically, colonoscopy is also an endoscopy (as is bronchoscopy) and I should say 'upper GI endoscopy' for the first one.

CLINICAL TIP 12: PULSES ARE GOOD FOR YOU

No, we haven't gone all wholemeal-vegetarian-sandal-wearing PC on you (who'd have thought baked beans would turn out to be a health food? Hopefully it'll be the pies next). I'm still unashamedly happy to ask anaemic patients if they have a normal diet or follow any bizarre fads like vegetarianism.[99]

This is to do with the other sort of pulse, a trio of tips reminding you that it is in fact good for you.

1 Temporal arteritis

It's good to have a pulse.

Including over the temporal artery. It's normal. The positive sign suggesting temporal arteritis is that the vessel is palpable, but the pulse is not. Lots of people get it round the wrong way.

2 Papilloedema

It's good to have a pulse.

Fundoscopy is, of course, nowadays normally performed with a CT scanner. But if you do find yourself looking through the right end of an ophthalmoscope at a blurred-ish disc, then a wee pulsation in the vein as it clambers out (in) from (to) the margin is a normal thing.

You can emphasise this by (lightly) pressing on the patient's eyeball (as an extra delicacy I often use the patient's eyelid to cushion the manoeuvre . . .) which should usually make the vein wince. If it *doesn't*, that *does* suggest papilloedema.

3 Life

It is good to have a pulse.

That whole not-being-dead thing. As a doctor, it's good to be able to take a pulse – since the world assumes that it's one thing even the worst doctor in the world can do. But while we were all taught endlessly how to find a radial pulse (thankfully not by the 'English' Royal College of Physicians since its logo shows it being done all wrong) no one actually teaches us how to feel a carotid pulse. And that's the one that your man-in-the-street knows is the one you use to check for life or death. Unfortunately most of us look for a carotid pulse based on what we've seen in films or on TV (copying our entire technique from what an actor thinks a

---

99 I have in the past admitted to enjoying a vegetarian lasagne – though the bits of beard do tend to get stuck in your teeth . . .

policeman thinks a doctor might do) and vaguely poke at one side or other of the neck.

What you should do is find the thyroid cartilage – the big sticky-out thing in the middle (laryngeal incisure . . . 'Adam's Apple' – less prominent in women, apparently[100]) – move an inch laterally and push medially into the natural tissue plane and slightly up (cephalically) and the pulse is there . . . or not.

CLINICAL TIP 13: MELAENA IS STICKY (AND BLOOD IS RED)

Yesterday's post-receiving ward round produced another patient who was diagnosed as 'a GI haemorrhage'. He had been 'vomiting blood' and had had 'melaena'.

The actual story he then gave me was that he had been bingeing on alcohol for some days, 1–2 bottles of vodka per day. Eating nothing. Eventually he felt sick and started to vomit. Dark stuff. 'Like bile' he called it, but had been told by doctors that this was blood. He found drinking more alcohol would settle things for a while . . . then the vomiting would return. He then developed diarrhoea. Runny brown stuff. Eventually he gave up on the vodka (it is, after all, entirely tasteless), still not eating anything, and moved on to . . . Guinness. Shortly after, the diarrhoea, whilst continuing, did change to being very dark runny stuff. The operative word is 'runny'.[101]

Melaena is sticky, gooey, thick, black stuff. It isn't runny. It's sticky. Runny diarrhoea is just that – diarrhoea – even if it's very dark. Diarrhoea. Not melaena (which is . . . sticky).

PS And Guinness is black.

---

100 I only learned this at the same time as Joey did (or was it Chandler?) in an episode of *Friends*.

101 I know this isn't the operative word. It's here an adjective, not a verb – but nobody uses that 'operative word' phrase literally. Or literarily. In fact, nobody uses it at all now . . . am I getting old? . . .

CLINICAL TIP 14: OCCAM'S RAZOR DOESN'T ALWAYS CUT THE MUSTARD

It's possible that many of you have no idea what Occam's Razor is – despite the fact you almost certainly use it daily in your diagnostic deliberations. It is often described – e.g. in Wikipedia (this week anyway) – as the 'wish to come up with a unifying diagnosis that will explain all of the patient's problems'. All very laudable. But it ain't perfect.

First of all, we should remember that William of Occam (Ockham) was not a physician, but a philosopher (day job – Franciscan monk) and his razor (not actually *his* razor,[102] but a mediaeval concept that was his favourite arguing technique – mine is *reductio ad absurdum*, but you've probably spotted that) referred not to medicine but to philosophical method. *Pluritas non est ponenda sine neccesitate* suggests we shouldn't invent lots of extra hypotheses or assumptions for a set of circumstances which can be explained by one hypothesis.[103] This became a tenet of scientific method, which was later applied to medical diagnostics. Searching for a unifying diagnosis is a reasonable principle, but it is not some fundamental which takes precedence over common sense. So while your patient with crushing chest pain, breathlessness, dizziness and a BP of 70/40 probably *has* had a heart attack (rather than an asthma attack . . . plus septicaemia plus Ménière's disease plus has just been hit on the sternum with a huge crushing-machine . . .) more chronic juxtapositions have to be viewed with extra care.

The human body is quite a complex piece of machinery. Over the period of a normal lifetime, it's amazing more things don't go seriously wrong. You wouldn't be happy flying across the Atlantic in an 80-year-old aeroplane – probably nor by an 80-year-old pilot, but you get my drift. Over the years, lots of different things are going to go wrong and it would be foolhardy to invariably attribute all of them to one 'disease' (unless that be Life itself). Take, for example . . .

(Those of you who have been avidly picking up clues to my personal approach to medicine – cynical, twisted, paranoid, but most of all *lazy* – will know what's coming next.)

. . . Psoriatic arthritis. (Aha! You all thought it was SLE . . . we'll get to that).

Psoriasis is a fairly common condition. Medical books will tell us it occurs in X% of the population (I'd love to fill in the value of X but I don't read

---

102 Any more than the needle belonged to Cleopatra.
103 As a monk he would presumably have been unimpressed by the later use of this principle to suggest that 'God' was an unnecessary fabrication to explain the laws of Nature.

medical books). Osteoarthritis, meantime, is outrageously common. It is pretty much a variant of normal. So when someone with psoriasis develops OA – don't go assuming they've got psoriatic arthritis. And if you do feel obliged to send them to the rheumatology clinic (where they'll ask us what to do about their skin 'cos not all of them will be having treatment for what they *do* have) then believe us when we say it isn't psoriatic arthropathy and don't keep referring to their 'psoriatic arthritis' in subsequent clinic letters to my supreme annoyance for ever and ever and ever . . .

We mentioned SLE, which is the other side of the same coin (as opposed to the other side of a totally different coin?). With psoriatic arthritis, the rheumatologist's hassle is that two separate problems are erroneously juxtaposed into one disease, so he has to see patients with some fiddly joint pains that otherwise wouldn't come near him. With SLE, the diagnosis is already made, and the problem is mainly for the patient in that every subsequent illness they have will be put down to the SLE – no matter how unlikely. It's well known that this disease has taken over from syphilis as 'the great pretender'. But whilst in the old days those people with symptoms of *other diseases* or *syphilis* had doctors who presumed they had the other disease until suddenly it turned out to be syphilis, nowadays their little-learning-is-a-dangerous-thing practitioners (trained by Prior-Based Learning) will assume it's their SLE until proven otherwise. Thus do odd rashes get referred to the rheumatologist (it was a reaction to an antibiotic) rather than a dermatologist, and pneumonias get treated with high-dose prednisolone.

Pawn's move thinking.

So . . . Occam's Razor.[104] Can point you in the right direction – but not always. Don't assume it does. Don't assume the liver disease is entirely due to the alcohol, the neuropathy is due to the diabetes, etc. It's a useful concept – but don't give it more kudos than it deserves. It is after all, basically a 400-year-old tip.

---

104 Why 'Razor'? No idea (why 'needle'?). It's not his own term (eighteenth-century, actually) and it doesn't seem to be some old word for 'principle'. Might just be to do with cutting away all the irrelevancies.

CLINICAL TIP 15: EVEN PARACELSUS NODS

This is a universally known tip – but generally misunderstood. When taking your favourite pulse – be it radial, carotid or (careful!) femoral – and you think it *might* be irregular, then we all know you should nod your head along with the pulse to help distingu– . . . except, you shouldn't.

If you nod your head with the pulse, you're just getting your head and neck muscles (. . . presumably . . . I've put that down in rather Cavalier fashion before checking with more knowledgeable colleagues that your head is in fact moved by neck muscles . . .) to do the job your fingertip was just doing. You are thus now asking the brain to decide if these muscles are contracting regularly – an almost identical task to deciding if a palpated pulse at your fingertips is regular. And whenever I make the nodding suggestion to students struggling with a tricky pulse, that's exactly what I watch them do – nod their heads in a slightly irregular fashion for a few seconds before announcing that the pulse is indeed regular.

What they should be doing is nodding in a *regular* rhythm based on the first couple of beats. So I force them to do so. When they find that the pulse they are feeling isn't fitting into this regular pattern, they suffer a brief annoy-ance at the beats not coming when expected. Their mouths open to speak, but they don't. Their brows furrow – should they change their nodding tempo, or change the patient's heart? Then their eyes light up as they realise . . . hey! . . . this pulse is *irregular*. It's atrial fibrillation![105]

---

105 Sinus arrhythmia can be excluded by not allowing the patient to breathe at any time throughout.

CLINICAL TIP 16: THE STERNAL ANGLE AND THE SECOND INTERCOSTAL . . .

I like to think that each of these tips has something for everyone. 'You're never too old to learn'[106] they say, and most tips are hopefully geared to make readers of all ages and levels at least think twice.

Not this one.

This tip is purely for medical students – 'cos real doctors really don't give a monkey's whether the apex beat is in the fifth or sixth intercostal space – or tenth, for that matter. They just slap their hand on the (usually) left side of the patient's chest[107] and vaguely note whether the apex beat is roughly where they expect it to be. Nobody actually counts down intercostal spaces. Amongst other reasons, this saves time explaining the manoeuvre to buxom barmaid-types (who've come along to the clinic as patients – not buxom barmaids *in situ*).

So this tip is for students. You will use it only once. When you count down to describe the position of the apex in your Finals.

Now, you all know ('cept the girl in today's teaching session) that you don't start from the clavicle, counting that as 'rib zero'. Nor do you start from the bottom, rupturing the patient's spleen whilst attempting to isolate a floating twelfth rib. You start at the sternal angle ('Angle of Louis' – as I like to term it for various reasons) – which is the angle between the manubrium and the sternum proper (NOT the sternal notch – which is the bit at the top of the sternum which is shaped rather like a notch) and absolutely *everybody* knows that the sternal angle is at the level of the second intercostal space . . . except IT ISN'T.

IT'S AT THE LEVEL OF THE SECOND RIB ITSELF.

I've described previously the fun (we don't get around much) for examiners watching the Finals' candidate find the sternal angle, move his/her finger across for the expected second intercostal space . . . only to find a *rib*! . . . major panic in the eyes . . . *is it the second or the third rib?*

(We don't really care, but it is fun.)

Now you won't have that dilemma.

---

106 Clearly not true. We're never too old to have something to learn, but actually learning anything I find increasingly impossible . . .

107 Most adroitly done, of course, by cardiologists – as that's where most guys keep their wallet.

CLINICAL TIP 17: SYNDROME OF INAPPROPRIATE ADH SECRETION IS LESS COMMON THAN BENDROFLUMETHIAZIDE

Snappy title.

And all you youngsters out there won't realise what an effort it was to write 'bendroflumethiazide' in big friendly letters – a drug I've known as 'bendrofluazide' (not that that would hugely help the snappiness) for 90% of my adult life.

A few years back, when some international drug authority-thingy decided they should rationalise the names of drugs worldwide, none of us took them seriously. But sure enough, lignocaine became 'officially' lidocaine, adrenaline became epinephrine,[108] and of course bendrofluazide ('BF') became bendroflumethiazide ('BF'). BFs. This has ruined the fun of patients' almost ritualistic mispronunciation of drugs ('I'm taking eighteen of those oxyhydrochloroquininininines[109] per day, Doctor'), since I now find myself hesitating before any witty correction (hey, maybe it *is* 'furosemide'[110]).

Globalisation of drug names does seem to make sense, but it is a bit tip-of-the-iceberg. It's not really going to help me get to grips with the patient's discharge letter from Warsaw General Hospital – any more than assuming we could all get on swimmingly in a hill-top restaurant in Montenegro as long as English and Montenegrin had the same words for the numbers one to ten. It'll just ensure the occasional bit makes sense. Like listening to traditional languages which have eschewed inventing 'modern' words for recent advances, and fallen back on the English. Watch any Japanese or Gaelic news programme to get the idea (. . . ayaaya ayaya aya computer aya ayaya yaay ay yaya *Strictly Come Dancing* ayayayaa . . .). To work properly, we'd have to build an entire medical Esperanto, everyone calling influenza 'la grippe', a heart attack 'Herzinfarkt', a headache 'glavobolju' (. . . might be Croatian . . .).

. . . where was I?

I remember.

When patients come in with Без леревода (Низкий натрий – oh, all right, *low sodium*), almost every 'receiving physician' assumes that inappropriate secretion of ADH is top of the differential diagnosis. They organise a CXR

---

108 One real annoyance was that *gentamicin* – a personal favourite anomaly – joined the other aminoglycosides in now being spelt with a 'y' *gentamycin*.

109 I think it's deliberate. Like the huge mispronunciation of the simplest of dishes in an Italian or French restaurant. A fear of looking as if you're trying your best yet failing leads to deliberate awfulness – like pronouncing the 'g' in 'Lasagne'.

110 Another particular annoyance. They changed the name to most patients' mistake!

(fair enough) plus serum and urine sodiums and osmolarities (also fair enough – though I for one am totally unable to interpret them), following up the 'normal' CXR report with tumour-marker requests and all-over CT scans and stuff. Meantime the patient's fluid intake is hugely restricted in an attempt 'to bring down their fluid volumes, thus increasing their sodium levels'.

All very well, except . . . nine times out of ten, the patient (particularly if elderly) is actually *dehydrated*, and *sodium depleted*, often simply from *being on diuretics* – or, of course, severe 'proljev'. What they need is the exact opposite of the above – a bit of fluid with a bit of salt, which, as it happens, is very readily available in handy individual plastic bags.

And how do you tell when it is the sIADH case? Well, all that urine/plasma sodiosmolarlity stuff does give you a proper answer, but they'll take days to come back, and an interim plan of withholding fluid from a potentially dehydrated patient doesn't sound ideal. Fortunately, there's a quick tip. Do the BP lying (after two minutes) and standing (immediately and after three minutes) and look for postural hypotension. If there is no suggestion of a postural drop, then sIADH becomes a genuine contender, but if the BP goes from 110/70 to 80/46 . . . maybe the patient needs some gentle saline (and a sit down) *but not too much too fast*. Care has to be taken with this. The point of the tip is to stop you spending the next three days waiting for lab results whilst actively dehydrating them further.

PS . . . did he say he was taking *eighteen?* . . .

CLINICAL TIP 18: DON'T GIVE UP ON LPs TOO EASILY[111]

When it comes to invasive investigations, I have to admit I'm a bit of a wuss. No point here in trying for some rock-hard street-cred when I keep dropping involuntary hints that I'm a rheumatologist. Cardiologists, respiratoriologists and gastroenterologists ram various-sized tubes up or down various-sized orifices and non-orifices before lopping off chunks of stuff or jabbing in electricity. What do rheumatologists do? Stick a tiny needle into a big skwudgy joint.

Arguably less invasive than venepuncture.

My eyes were opened to this at a talk by a local orthopod who opined that – providing you first draw back to check you're not in a blood vessel or the heart – there really isn't very much damage you can do to *anything* when you're aspirating or injecting a joint – as long as you never inject against resistance. So I looked up all the books and pamphlets and diagrams showing you where exactly to insert the needle, and at what angle, for the various joint injections and realised . . . these techniques were elementary in the extreme. They pretty much used the same route my five-year-old daughter would take if you asked *her* to stick a needle in somebody's ankle or knee (I baulk at suggesting my son. He'd banjax the needle trying to go straight through the patella. Still, he's only 25).

Arguably less *difficult* than venepuncture, then. You don't need to plump up a leg with a tricky tourniquet just to find a knee.

It makes sense really. And confirms I didn't go into medicine because I was the sort of person who liked to hurt people or damage them (if I was, I'd have become a hit man for the Mafia, or a physio). I'm not a big fan of putting in chest drains, pacemakers, even urinary catheters – though at least then I know where I'm going.

So . . . I *totally* understand that when anyone's doing a lumbar puncture and they've done that find-the-line-across-the-iliac-crests bit[112] and they know they can go into the inter-spinous process space either above or below this line . . . they will always try the one below. But when this fails (as it often does), you've got to try the one above. The number of times I'm told that an LP 'failed' and they couldn't get CSF and then you go see the patient and the only LP attempt(s) are below the iliac-crest line is . . . (no satisfyingly impressive way to end this ranting sentence; should have thought ahead) high.

---

111 Not an anti-CD rant – though I do feel the loss of two-sided vinyl has reduced the elegance of track-ordering. Now you just start with any good ones and gradually drift into rubbish.

112 '. . . that's because it's an *imaginary* line, Professor . . . and I was meaning *at the back*.'

To be honest, a good case could be made for missing out entirely the 'one-below' shot and go straight for the 'one-above' – but probably not by a wuss like me.

CLINICAL TIP 19: ANTI-DIABETES DRUGS ARE INTERESTING

OK. They're not. But I was looking for a title that would capture the imagination. And one of them does have a couple of interesting features.

Metformin.

Hopefully, when this is published, metformin will still be a diabetic staple and won't have been superseded by something called gliptizonohumoglitizonimab or somesuch which stops your gut absorbing glucose *plus* stops your liver making glucose from other substances, *plus* turns any glucose already in your body (though . . . how on earth did that get there?) into an inert polymer that lines your arteries and viscera with a soothing Teflon coating, reducing heart attacks, stroke, cancer and more than likely preventing global warming . . .

. . . So it will still be of some use to you to remember . . .

1 *Never* blame metformin for blackouts or funny turns. Metformin does *not* cause hypoglycaemia. It works by enhancing the effects of insulin (and a few other things), not by releasing extra insulin, so how could it cause hypoglycaemia? No-way-no-how. That's why it *doesn't*.

2 *Always* blame metformin for diarrhoea.

OK. Not always. It's never always (and, of course, never never usually, most of the time). But metformin does very often cause loose bowel motions and can cause severe diarrhoea (even steatorrhoea).

The endocrinologist who gave me this double-tip (a blatant attempt to shake off the image of the unhelpful endocrinology stereotype who wouldn't give you the time of day[113]) also gave me (it's habit-forming once you start) his example of a 50-year-old woman whose diarrhoea and weight loss was chased up and down (literally) by the surgeons who eventually asked him to see her. He stopped her metformin and it all got better. Mark up another one to the phys-i-cians . . .

. . . except . . . the reason he was asked to see her was that the eighty-fourth investigation – a CT scan of abdomen – had shown an adrenal

---

113 They apparently also 'wouldn't piss on you if you were on fire' but, to be fair, I'd put that down to their old-world genteel courtesy rather than genuine ill-will.

mass, which turned out to be an adenoma . . . which as it happens was causing the diabetes for which she had blithely been given metformin by the endocrinologists in the first place . . . and had now been spotted early on a CT that was only done because . . . nobody knew *not* to look . . .

And the moral of the story is that not all stories have a moral . . . or maybe they have more than one moral . . . or a whole complex moral structure (Tip 19 vs. *The Bible*).

PS Sulphonylureas such as glipizide, gliclazide, etc. (which work by prompting the release of extra [pro]insulin) *do* cause hypoglycaemia. Sometimes severe. Sometimes long-lasting. So if you see a non-diabetic patient who's accidentally taken them or overdosed, don't send them away with casual advice to have a cup of tea. They need to be looked after.

SDS

CLINICAL TIP 20: STATUS EPILEPTICUS STARTS AT 20 MINUTES

OK. Hands up . . . what do you do when a patient with known epilepsy starts to 'have a seizure'[114] – no . . . be honest. *You* don't put them into the recovery position. The nurses do that. What do *you* do? Absolutely! Give them intravenous diazepam . . .

. . . now tell me why? . . .

No. IV diazepam is a treatment for status epilepticus – which, as we all know, is 'seizure activity going on for more than 15 . . . 20 . . . or 30 minutes (depending on your source of wisdom) without recovery'. Worth remembering that recurrent seizures without full recovery of consciousness between them also fits[115] the bill. But meantime lets get back to why you are giving diazepam after two minutes? Can't answer, eh? 'Cos the two reasons are slightly embarrassing – 'cos they are:
  1 You don't like to look as if you are not doing anything.
  2 The nurses are telling you to give it.

Two tips in one, really.
  1 Sometimes it's right to not do anything. Look after the patient, but use drugs only if they are actually required. In this case, only if there is no

114 Not supposed to say 'fit', though its use as a verb here would save a lot of time.
115 It's OK here.

recovery after 10–15 minutes. People have seizures at home all the time. A hospital bed is arguably a safer place to have one. So why rush to abort this one using pharmaceuticals?
2 Don't do something just because somebody else thinks you should.

CLINICAL TIP 21: DIAZEPAM IS BETTER AT ABOLISHING SEIZURES THAN PREVENTING THEM

Not to say that it doesn't act to prevent them. Benzodiazepines do have a major anticonvulsant effect – though their tendency to stop working after a time (tachyphylaxis or habituation or something) limits their use as long-term anticonvulsants. They are sometimes used in short bursts such as in 'catamenial epilepsy', where some young women tend to get clusters of seizures around the time of the menses.

In the acute 'status epilepticus' scenario, IV diazepam will abolish the seizure activity approximately 95% of the time – but it will recur in up to 50% of cases. Phenytoin, meantime, will be arguably less effective at abolishing the seizure, but arguably more effective at preventing further episodes.

The upshot of this was apparently unclear to most people when I attended an epilepsy conference years ago. In a big fancy hall incorporating what were state-of-the-art interactive facilities – a little box with buttons marked ABCD at each seat (I suppose these days you scan your mobile phone across your forehead). When we were all asked whether we use diazepam or phenytoin or two other bizarre choices in acute status, the ensuing histogram (in colour!) showed that only two of us had suggested phenytoin. The chairman asked if either of these eccentrics would be brave enough to show their hand and explain their choice. The more eccentric of them did – I pointed out that I was in the fortunate position (at the back – where else?) of having empty seats beside me so I could press both buttons – as I would always give both. Diazepam to eradicate the seizure, *plus* IV phenytoin (15–18 mg/kg *slowly*) to help prevent recurrence.

I like to think that that day I influenced the worldwide ILAE's[116] approach to status epilepticus. The ILAE doesn't.

---

116 International League Against Epilepsy. Honest. Not an Arthur Conan Doyle fabrication.

CLINICAL TIP 22: WHEN YOUR BOSS MAKES A MISTAKE . . . TELL THEM

This tip differs from Clinical Tips 2 and 3 since it concerns the boss of your own team. A trickier situation.

Here's a funny thing about aircraft crashes (bet you thought there *wasn't* one). They're more likely to happen when the boss pilot is flying the plane than when the co-pilot is. Seems odd, but then people realised that when one guy is 'just' flying the thing, the other guy is watching out for any problems – be they other aircraft, instrument malfunctions, ground-to-air missiles, or indeed mistakes or misjudgements by the pilot. Not only would perhaps boss-man's extra experience make him better at this, it definitely makes him better at telling the other guy.

Think of it as dad teaching his son to drive:

> Dad: You're going a bit fast for that corner coming up, son.
> Son: OK, Dad. [SLOWS DOWN]

Alternatively, same speed, same corner, dad at wheel:

> Son: Er, Dad . . . this seems . . . maybe a bit . . . [THINKS: Oh, I suppose
>   he knows what he's doing] . . .
> Dad: What was that, son? . . . Whooo-ooops!

That's how we got all the 'gosh it does look quite icy out there on the wing' stuff from the co-pilot a few years back instead of a 'Whoah!!! We can't take off!' shortly before an overloaded-with-ice plane went into the Potomac River.

Ward rounds are dangerous places too. People can come to harm if mistakes are made. Not so much for the guys on our side of the fence (unless the ward round's headed up by a particularly bad-assed orthopod). We're quite safe. So if it's difficult for a co-pilot whose own life is in jeopardy to tell the boss he might be doing something wrong, we can see how tricky it might be for the junior doctor, with less personal investment.

But it's gotta be done.

Whether it's 'is there a reason for the high dose?' or 'did we mention the patient was on warfarin?' (when you know you did), you must find some way to stick your nose in if your boss is doing something wrong. I am here assuming it's important to the patient. 'Those shoes really don't go with that top, Chief' isn't recommended.

And you can't just sneak back and rectify things later.

a)   You might forget/be waylaid.
b)   Your boss has to learn not to do it next time.

You don't need to be rude, loud or embarrassing – but you need to get it done.

All of which makes me wonder: would we be best always having the junior do the ward round with the consultant tagging along as wing-man?

CLINICAL TIP 23: A HAEMOGLOBIN IS USELESS WITHOUT AN MCV

Maybe this is an overstated personal foible. Most of my stuff is. But when a junior tells me a recently admitted patient's haemoglobin is '8.5' I immediately want to know what the MCV is (as well as the units for the haemoglobin – if that's g/L maybe we should panic). I want to have some sort of idea what is going on with the patient, rather than the simple information that they are anaemic.

In fact, maybe I should claim that I'd rather have the MCV without the haemoglobin than the other way round. The haemoglobin level does, after all, only tell you the grade of the problem, rather than what the problem might be. I'd rather you told me the name of the bug that was found in a guy's sputum than supply a colorimetric analysis saying just how green it was. A low oxygen result without the CO_2 level is similarly unhelpful . . .

I think the investigations you would carry out on someone with an MCV of 110 will not depend at all on what the actual haemoglobin is. It's irrelevant. In fact, I need to upgrade the tip, give it a bit of controversy.

CLINICAL TIP 23a: DON'T MEASURE HAEMOGLOBIN, JUST THE MCV[117]

---

117 What do you mean *what about treating people and making them better?*

CLINICAL TIP 24: ALWAYS CHECK HAEMATINICS BEFORE GIVING A TRANSFUSION

Makes sense.

Back to the old police-work analogy. This time, not disturbing the crime scene.

> Detective: Thank you, Constable. I'll take over from here . . . mmmmm . . . there are some footprints here leading towards . . .
> Constable: Er . . . those are mine, Chief.
> Detective: . . . OK . . . [BENDS DOWN] . . . mmmmm . . . looks like they moved the body. The lividity in the . . .
> Constable: Er . . . that was us, Boss. The light wasn't too good for the photographs, so we . . .
> Detective: [GLOWERS BRIEFLY. RETURNS TO BODY] Aha! These gunshot wounds. No bleeding. Looks like the killers first strangled their victim, then shot him to make it look . . .
> Constable: Er . . . that was us, Boss. He was dead anyway, so I thought – no harm in using him for a bit of pistol practice . . .

Anaemia isn't a complete diagnosis. You want to know what caused the anaemia. As with everything else, the patient's story can give you a clue, but can also lead you up the garden path. Vegetarianism isn't a dead giveaway if they're folate deficient.

For a start, you want to know what kind of anaemia, and you find out from the blood film (MCV, retics, RDW, etc.) and haematinics (iron studies, folate, B12). Since all this evidence will be washed away by a blood transfusion, always take off blood for these before transfusing (and maybe haptoglobins). And don't just ask somebody to do it, or write it down; make sure it's done. Otherwise you end up waiting for the patient to become anaemic again (whereupon someone else will transfuse them without checking).

You don't need to wait for the results, just make sure they will happen – though if the transfusion itself is not urgent, it will often be best to wait . . . in fact . . .

CLINICAL TIP 24a: DON'T RUSH TO TRANSFUSE SOMEONE UNLESS IT'S AN EMERGENCY

CLINICAL TIP 25: ALWAYS FOCUS ON THE PART OF THE STORY WHICH DOESN'T FIT

Last receiving day, I was told about an old lady who'd been brought in. Radiotherapy for pelvic malignancy had left her with 'radiation proctitis' and recurrent severe anaemia from the blood loss. She'd come in again with a haemoglobin of eight. The junior mentioned that her story *didn't actually include any rectal bleeding or melaena*.

What's the MCV?	Dunno. [CTip 23]
Is she transfused yet?	Yes. [CTip 24a]
Did you do the haematinics?	No. [CTip 24+]
Why not?	They were done last time. [CTip 5]
What were they then?	Dunno.

We found the MCV: 98 fL. Not iron deficient. We took her story. 'Proctitis' causing eight bowel movements per day at worst. No blood, no melaena. Conceivably this, or ongoing malignancy is causing a chronic-disease anaemia, but it's not causing blood loss or iron deficiency so this lady needs a few more investigations. My guess, myelodysplasia (wrong, of course).

If there's some little glitch in the glib scenario offered up as a diagnosis by others (indeed, by yourself) then focus on that glitch.

Career Tips

It might seem odd to take career advice from someone who spent 47 years as a registrar and who once (at a job interview) replied to the Professor of Clinical Pharmacology's question about measuring a drug's potency, with 'surely you mean efficacy?',[118] but . . .

. . . Actually, it does seem odd.

CAREER TIP 1: IF YOU'RE GOING TO FLASH, FLASH HARD

Before you ask, it's a cricketing analogy.

If the ball is whizzing past the outside of your wicket and you vaguely poke at it, then it's quite likely to nick the edge of your bat, zip into the keeper's gloves, and you're *out* 'caught behind'. Conventional wisdom is that if you are going to prod in such an uncontrolled way, then you might as well have a wild swing at the thing since if the ball does clip your bat it'll fly off wildly in any direction making it a) less likely you'll get caught and b) more likely you might pick up a run or two. Hence: IF YOU'RE GOING TO FLASH (*out-side off-stump*), FLASH HARD.

The medical tip concerns dealing with the exasperating patient who via heart-sinkness, vagueness, uselessness or just plain nastiness eventually pings

---

118 I don't actually remember this. But its veracity is assured by an ex-classmate who was on the other side of the table. Yes. A senior registrar interview down south and I am being interviewed by an old classmate who's already an established consultant. Maybe you should read *his* Career Tips.

you off the end of your tether prompting you to give them a mouthful. And the tip is to make this mouthful so impossibly awful that no one (including any GMC committee) in their right mind (if a GMC committee can have a right mind) could possibly believe for a moment that it could have come from your lips.

Think about it:

> That doctor said I was a malingerer and there's nothing wrong with me.

> He can't say that! Sue him.

. . . or try . . .

> That doctor said I was a lazy good-for-nothing mother-f***ing sh**-bag son-of-a-*!$@* who should be put down like the rest of the vermin in my family so he's ordered a Hit on me with MI6.

> . . . er . . . really? . . .

It was difficult to categorise this tip – other than as extremely useful. Clearly, it's 'Cynical', but I thought perhaps I should put it in under 'Career' . . . though I wouldn't necessarily insist a young recruit try it out to further one. Indeed I wondered if maybe the tip was a bit too . . . postmodern . . . in its outlook to be included at all. But we get back to the cricketing analogy. If you're going to flash, flash hard. It's a big 'if' (though the italics, paradoxically, did sort-of make it look smaller). The real trick is not to be tempted in the first place by the bowl just outside off-stump. Just bide your time, and watch the ball pass harmlessly by . . .[119]

DR

---

119 Have just realised. Patients could now claim I've said the most ridiculous things about them and my 'that's a bit unlikely' defence has just been blown out the water since I've shown my awareness of it (cf. *Time to Kill*: J Grisham). It would be better if this book never gets published (cf. *Time to Kill*: J Grisham).

CAREER TIP 2: TIPS ARE JUST TIPS

They're no substitute for understanding or common sense.

Spent yesterday examining for the membership.

Presented with 'rheumatoid hands', three out of five candidates requested (no . . . demanded . . .) a pillow. Having spent, for the last 30 years, half my waking hours (and a disturbing proportion of the sleeping ones) as a rheumatologist, and never having myself employed said object for such a function, I had to ask 'why?' . . . to be supplied with amazingly vague 'more-comfortable-for-the-patient' chaff. Since I presumed we didn't plan standing idly by watching the patient rest her hands, and would instead be picking them up, making them do various functional manoeuvres, and indeed squeezing them TO SEE HOW SORE THAT WAS . . . I didn't quite see what difference it would make doing all of this six inches above a nice soft pillow.

But then I realised. This was *a tip*. Either they'd all gone on the same course, or a big bunch of courses were teaching the same thing (which did briefly panic me that *I* was the black sheep until a co-examiner-rheumatologist backed me up).

I later realised it was the same three who identically rounded off the hand examination by grabbing their stethoscopes and yanking at the lady's blouse, vowing to check her lungs for fibrosis ('you get that in rheumatoid arthritis . . .'). My pointing pointedly at the other onlooking 'short cases' in the entirely open ward did manage to dissuade two of the candidates, though we had to physically restrain one enthusiast ('Aw . . . come on! – they've all got eye drops in anyways . . .'). Nobody asked to feel for a spleen (Felty's), or feet for peripheral neuropathy (just as well . . . they do have only five minutes), so clearly the listen-to-the-chest thing was . . . *a tip*.

Tips are not intrinsically bad things (though never trust them if they're described as 'Top') and the above examples aren't too distressing. But you can't let them take the place of normal thinking. All three candidates also asked – with regard to 'pincer function' – for the patient to do up a button. Her clothes didn't include a button (she had rheumatoid arthritis!) to which their reaction can only be described as . . . *annoyance*. One entirely gave up the idea of assessing pincer grip. His tip-withdrawal paralysis was even more clamant when it came to the scleroderma patient.[120] He volunteered checking for microstomia and asked the patient to put three fingers in her own mouth. As her fingers had severe flexion contractures (she had scleroderma! What planet do these tips come from?), this was a non-starter. He again gave up:

---

120 No we didn't have two rheumatology patients just so I would have the slightest clue. The scleroderma was 'skin'. I don't pick 'em.

So . . . does she have microstomia?

I don't know.

Why not?

Her fingers are flexed . . . the test doesn't work . . . you should be able to get three fingers . . .

But . . . she's still got a mouth?

?!

Well . . . is it small?

. . . don't know . . . can't tell . . . her fingers are flexed and . . .

Tips are just tips. You should always know the idea behind them. And you should always think of them as 'extras' – ways for things to be done that bit better. If they don't work, you have to go back to first principles. So it does help if you know some.

CAREER TIP 3: USE THE TIE CARD FLEXIBLY (*À LA* JAN 2008)

When and where to wear a tie?

As the world slowly changes – eventually even for doctors (famous for being Cconservative with both '*c*'s) – and the answer moves inexorably from 'always' to 'never', you need some indications of current appositeness (always remembering that this is through the eyes of a 50-year-old who uses bogus words like appositeness).

Being interviewed for job	Yes.
Interviewing for job	Yes (unless going for that raffish cool-guy-around-campus look. Though be careful if this is obviously because of cute interviewee).
Being interviewed for job	Yes! I told you. Even if you *are* going for that raffish cool-guy- . . .
Doing clinic	Yes. It looks and feels right. And if it does spread diseases, nobody has got round to blaming docs yet as it's not so obvious that you've given somebody a disease if you let them go home and spend a dangerously normal life for a few days.[121]

(continued)

---

121 Since writing, we have all been commanded not to wear a tie at clinic. Drat. Many of the above advices may be superseded by rules. Watches too now. This whole tip ruined . . . can't be bothered writing another one. Maybe I could make it 'use the wedding ring card flexibly'.

Doing *private* ward round	Yes.
Or clinic	Yes.
Speaking to relatives	Yes.
Speaking to relatives whose relative is suffering from *C. diff.* or *MRSA*	No.
Doing surgical ward round/clinic	Yes. Surgeons are much more Cconservative than physicians but have a Ddilemma. No-tie fits with the we're-all-real-men-here ethos, but a tie does help mark them out from other corner-boys. Wear one 'meantime'.
In theatre	No. To be fair, I think the infection-control people have got this one right.
At the theatre	No.
At the pictures	No.
In the pictures, e.g. when wooing female lead in RomCom	No. The guy wearing a tie is always gonna lose out, even if already engaged to heroine, and even if the other guy is as unattractive as Tom Hanks.
Cooking dinner	No. Even if you love Tie Cuisine.[122]
Having sex	Depends . . .

I think I've lost track of my remit here . . .

CAREER TIP 4: ALWAYS ASK THE PATIENT IF IT'S OK TO SPEAK ABOUT THEM TO A RELATIVE

You see it all the time. Somebody phones up to say they're Mrs Bloggs's sister and how's she doing? . . . and what tests have you done? . . . and when's she getting out? – and the nurse or doctor just sits there and tells them. If you were cuddled up on your sofa, watching this in some conspiracy movie, you'd be screaming at the TV, *'Don't tell them . . . No! **Don't** tell them . . .'*

    Now . . . I'm not saying this woman's sister (if, indeed, it *is* her sister . . .) wants to know how long she's laid up for so she can go rob the house, or find out what room she's in so she can dress up as a doctor using a handy white coat she'll find in the linen cupboard and sneak in and finish her off with an intravenous wallop of insulin/potassium or with a nice soft pillow that an MRCP candidate would kill their granny to get their (rheumatoid) hands on . . . I'm just saying THIS IS NONE OF HER BUSINESS.

---

122 . . .What?

That is, until the patient says it's her business.

This isn't just part of my doesn't-actually-exist-honest anti-relatives ven-detta. I have genuinely seen cases where a doctor/nurse has chatted to a patient's 'sister in London . . . I'm a nurse myself' or 'friend in Canada' and the patient has been thoroughly non-pleased. And rightly so. This is a clear breach of confidentiality.

When a patient's relative (and how do you know it *is* a relative?) or friend (in which case I'd seriously consider not talking to them even if the patient says you can) wants you to tell them about a patient's illness – whether it be over the phone or face-to-face – you go ask the patient if that is OK.

It's right at the confidentiality level.

It's right at the James Bond level.

It's right at the what's-in-it-for-me level. There's a bonus, you see. Hands up all of you who *like* talking to patient's relatives? I thought as much . . .'cos there's always the chance the patient will tell you not to bother.

CAREER TIP 5: TRY A BIT OF CROSS-GUESSING

Ever wondered why every male nurse you see is already a 'sister'. Or why every female orthopaedician is already a consultant (despite looking like it'd take them half a week to saw through Wayne Rooney's metacarpal)? It's because they've followed this tip (not necessarily consciously – it *is* possible for some svelte Sloane debutante to be seduced by the beer-swilling, rugger-and-golf, hammer-and-chisel world that is orthopaedic surgery – but most likely it has been an astute career move) which is – *choose a specialty where your sex is less than adequately represented.*[123]

Think about it.

A girl and four blokes go for an orthopaedic job. Already she stands out like a healthy thumb. Subliminally the interviewer's choice is between giving the job to the girl or to one of the boys – so already she's improved her odds from one-in-five to a straight evens bet. And there are good reasons to choose her. A woman would bring a new dimension to any such unit. A balanced . . . caring approach . . . patient-oriented . . .

Meantime a boy looking for a job in one of the female-dominated specialties such as geriatrics or (ahem!) rheumatology can bring all those male attributes that will give him an advantage over females which I can't mention

---

123 Could have made that less bizarre by using 'gender', but I have this pedantic streak that only lets me use that word etymologically.

here as that would be sexist (in the same way that mentioning lots of female advantages isn't . . .).[124]

And once you've got your consultant job, it just keeps on giving. It's easier to get noticed. Anyone organising an area meeting looking for a couple of speakers from a group of nine men and one woman, or vice versa, will know what's needed to give the meeting some balance.

The only trick is to spot where these lopsided specialties will arise in the future – since the demographics are always changing, particularly when people start to play the odds. Wouldn't be the first time someone wanting to be the only woman in gynaecology made their move just when lots of women go into gynaecology. But at least the uncertainty does give some justification for the tip's clippy title.

CAREER TIP 6: WITH FEATHERS ALL FLUFFY AND BROWN . . .

No one would want to spend their entire life stacking shelves at Safeway's (cf. famous Government negotiator's comment[125] back in the good old Thatcher days[126] of the internal market that 'if we think of the NHS as a giant commercial corporation such as Safeway then the consultants would be the guys stacking the shelves'). But you don't spend your life stacking shelves. You move onwards and upwards until you're the Top Banana who can get rid of the more threateningly ambitious shelf stackers with ultra-imaginative catch-phrases like 'you're fired'.

Caterpillars get to become butterflies. Ugly ducklings get to be beautiful swans.

So when you're looking to pick a career path, try to see past the life of the 'junior' in any particular specialty (e.g. paediatrics where it can be miserable – though mainly because of the senior paediatricians). Watch what the consultant's life consists of, not the junior's, since a consultant is what you'll spend most of your time as – particularly these days when run-through training takes about a fortnight.

And whilst I'm bitterly battering on at my favourite hobby-horse (next to

---

124 E.g. we can't say that a few more guys in the specialty might make people take it seriously . . .
125 The comment's famous, not the negotiator.
126 It's the days that were good,[126a] not . . .
126a Poetic licence for the sake of comedy.

mixed metaphors) of the modern fad for changes-for-no-reason, don't forget that it works both ways. These days, the junior's life just might be easier than that of the consultant.

There once was a pretty tadpole
With . . .

HD

CAREER TIP 7: DON'T HAVE AN AFFAIR WITH YOUR SECRETARY

Obviously, there are lots of people you shouldn't have an affair with – no matter how attractive they, and indeed you, are. Since many of these are at the level of being *rules* of Ethics and all that sort of stuff (patients, patients' relatives, students, *your* relatives . . .), then it would seem a bit superfluous to mention them here as 'tips'.

Secretaries have, however, not been chosen simply because they're the most likely candidates after the absolute *no-nos* and therefore the most likely relative *no-nos* – which would in fact be nurses. No. Secretaries are different from all the above because you shouldn't have an affair with them *even if nobody will ever find out* (oops. It is possible that that's generally considered true for at least some of the others . . . but it's always been my approach that the reason you don't have an affair with a patient is in case somebody finds out you're having an affair, and similarly you don't have an affair with a nurse in case somebody finds out she's a nurse . . .). Secretaries are bad news because, once you slip into the traditional boy–girl role-playing:

1 She'll[127] never do any typing for you (even if you dress up).
2 You won't be able to crack jokes even in the workplace without getting the eye-rolling treatment.
3 Who would you get to pick out her Christmas present?

127 Yes, the secretary is the female. Otherwise they won't earn enough.

CAREER TIP 8: DON'T GIVE/GET YOUR WIFE A JOB IN YOUR UNIT

Self-evident.

If you do break this rule, then NEVER break Career Tip 7.

CAREER TIP 9: ALWAYS TELL THE TRUTH AT INTERVIEWS

Not everyone's advice – but my thinking goes like this.

You tell lies at an interview ('Yes, I've always wanted to be a geriatrician, ever since I was very little, and Edinburgh is such a wonderful city.') and you get the job. Hurrah. Well done. Now:

1 You've just been dishonest. Morally dubious. Ethically worrying (when it comes to the 'probity' section in your first appraisal, you'll get all embarrassed when your appraiser tells you what the word means). Of course, these days moral reprehensibility is arguably no acceptable reason to put you off a particular course of action[128] – so let's see if I can convince you with . . .

2 Psychologically, you'll be haunted by the worry you got the job under false pretences (basically, because you did) and by subsequent pangs of unworthiness. There's a certain satisfaction in achieving something you want, and surely this is reduced if you have done it deviously? Apparently, at games, etc. I'm outrageously competitive. It surprises many people, therefore, when they realise that I never cheat.[129] Maybe I just don't play sports /games at a high enough level. Why call my pal's cross-court volley out, meaning I've won the match, since there'd be no real satisfaction in that win? But make it Wimbledon . . .

So I suppose I must bow to the possibility that anyone who does tell lies at interviews may think the gains are so major that they are happy to reconcile themselves to that, which leaves me with trump card . . .

3 You are now working for/with someone who wants to work over/with someone who would have honestly given the answer you gave to the question, i.e. *not* you. You are not the person they think you are, or the person they want. A problem if it's your boss, but arguably worse if it's your colleague, if this is your ultimate consultant interview and you'll spend the rest of your life working with these people.

A bit like telling your prospective spouse yes-you-want-children when

---

128 Otherwise so much in life would be rendered impossible – from running a bank to invading a country.

129 Cf. standard tip re 'never say *never* in medicine'

you don't, or no-you-don't when you do – because it's what they wanted to hear.

And if you are just telling lies at the interview so that you can get this job for a short time before leaving them in the lurch to go on to the one you really want in any case and so none of the above really applies to you . . . I'd prefer it if you read someone else's book.

CAREER TIP 10: ALWAYS ANSWER 50:50 QUESTIONS IN WRITTEN EXAMS

This is perhaps losing some usefulness, as exams such as the MRCP make less and less use of the true–false format, but by the time this book is published fashion's tide should have turned again.

I've never understood why people were so scared of 'losing a mark' in true–false questions. As long as you don't lose two marks for a mistake vs. gaining one for a correct answer, then the odds are clearly stacked in favour of guessing.

Let's say there are 300 questions. There are 200 where you 'know' the answer. What's your plan with the other 100? Well, if you got a monkey to guess them all, then on average he[130] will get 50 right and 50 wrong – for a net score of zero, which will not alter the score out of the first 200. If you refuse to guess at the last 100, you are saying you expect to do worse than the monkey. Surely, using your general medical knowledge over 100 questions, that will not be the case?[131] So guess them all. If you get 51 right and 49 wrong – that's two extra marks (which you might need – are you absolutely sure that you got every one of the first 200 right?).

'But,' I hear you cry, 'every time I guess, I get it wrong!'

Balderdash!

What you really mean is every time you find out you got one wrong, you'd guessed that one. Probably true, but not the same thing. A lot of the ones you got right, you also guessed. You see, when you guess an answer and it turns out to be right, your psyche interprets this as something you sort-of knew . . . but when your guess turns out to be wrong, then that *was* a guess and you're so unlucky that you're always wrong if you guess. So if you go through an

---

130 A female monkey will refuse to take part in anything so pointless.
131 Liability waiver. Please note all arguments in this book relate to medical exams and cannot necessarily be extrapolated to, for example, FRCS.

exam answering 20 questions you're not sure of, and 14 are right, you'll only remember the other six as the 'guesses'.

So guess them all.

. . . Actually, my advice is not to guess them *all*. Absolute random guessing cannot be good for the soul. My advice is this:

➤ If you are unsure whether to go True or leave it . . . *True*
➤ If you are unsure whether to go False or leave it . . . *False*
➤ If you are unsure whether to go True or False or leave it . . . *leave it*

PS Please note whilst this is my advice for passing exams, it does not sit easily with my ethos of being a doctor. Doctors shouldn't really guess, and it's unfortunate that such a technique does help them through their training. Personally I would advocate the marking system I lightly suggested above – two marks off for a wrong answer, making guessing unattractive. However, I would couple this with the abandonment of abstruse, small-print, triple negative and down-right-daft questions.

PPS Notice the 'written' in the title. When a clinical examiner gives you a 50:50 choice, then you might find it reasonable to prevaricate. I used to take great glee in asking juniors five 50:50s about heart attacks.

1 Would you rather have an anterior or an inferior infarct?
2 Which of those two is more likely to cause conduction defects?
3 Which is more dangerous, Mobitz or Wenckebach second-degree heart block?
4 Which of those two is now called 'Mobitz 1'? [This was some time ago.]
5 You are leaving the hospital after recovering from your heart attack. Your pal who was on the team looking after you tells you that you had an episode . . . either of atrial fibrillation or of ventricular fibrillation . . . which would you rather he said?

(See Appendix 1 for answers).

If I managed to get the SHO/whatever to get all five wrong (it's designed to, if you give them the answers as you go) then I would point to the coin-tossing scenario in Statistics Tip 2 and declare them statistically less smart than a monkey (as I must have suspected all along . . . otherwise it wouldn't be significant . . . two-tailed monkeys and all that).

CAREER TIP 11: PATIENTS FROM YOUR HOME TOWN DON'T PAY THEIR BILLS

(Private: don't tell anyone)

In the interests of this book appealing to all species of doctor, I thought I'd include a tip for those indulging in the practice that dare not speak its name.

One of the drawbacks of private medicine is dealing with patients who don't pay their bills. And it goes against the grain for doctors to chase them up in the courts or send the boys out after them. Not just because they're likely to know bigger boys than the doctor does. It just feels . . . wrong. A bit unseemly. Not the done thing.

So the plan is to spot the likely fare-dodgers before you let them on the bus. And one helpful pointer I've noticed is: patients from your home town (or area) don't pay their bills.

The reason is unclear. It may be the infamous 'I kent his faither' Scottishism of not taking a local lad seriously (cf. McCassandra). Alternatively they may feel they are due some special consideration. So I canvassed some colleagues for their views.

They'd never come across the phenomenon.

Signals' check on that title:

Patients from *my* home town don't pay their bills.

CAREER TIP 12: TURN UP FOR BEDSIDE TEACHING

When I were a lad . . . we used to spend the first two years at medical school learning about science. Chemistry, Biology, Physiology . . . daft really. Sitting up all night trying to solve Entropy equations whilst your social life falls to pieces . . . writing essays on 'how birds are adapted for flight' (apparently feathers are very warm and very, very light[132]) when you really should be attacking pterodactyls in Dungeons and Dragons . . . looking up case histories trying to find one where a patient's presenting complaint was 'it's my ATPase, doctor' . . . All seems totally useless now – though you can still win coffee-room money betting on how many ovaries a chaffinch has.

These days, of course, there's none of that. Right from the off, it's all to do with medicine. Real medicine.

---

132 So what's the Tog value of titanium, then?

So how come final-year students, or even first-year doctors, look as though they've never actually seen a patient before? Simple concepts we take for granted repeatedly flash 'Breaking News!' frowns across their angelic faces. In last week's bedside teaching (genuinely), 'pulse deficit' cropped up (for any orthopaedic surgeon who's picked up this book by accident,[133] that's the phenomenon in atrial fibrillation where the radial pulse has fewer beats than the heart itself, as they don't all 'get through').

No one had any idea what it was – and my prompting produced the suggestion that the left ventricle might have *fewer* beats than the pulse at the wrist.

Why is this? (i.e. students not knowing stuff, not why does atrial fibrillation cause you to have a pulse deficit which is just a simple matter of not being able to feel weak pulses).

I think it's a paradoxical effect (though, to be fair, I think everything is) where, by keeping us young students from any clinical medicine for two years, we were so dead keen to get into the wards and see patients that we turned up, ready and focused, and learned a lot more. Even the guys who skipped most lectures and tutorials (and later suffered hugely when managing ketoacidosis because they couldn't remember what happened to the second NADPH in the Krebs cycle) would turn up at all the bedside teaching. Four or five medical students and a doctor sitting around the bed of an accommodating (and hopefully keen) patient, having a relaxed time. What could be better than that? Every day of the week at 9.15 am. You got used to it. It didn't necessarily feel like you were learning anything. The same things would crop up, punctuated by nice moments like the bronchitic man who complained of a 'wheezle' in his chest, and a colleague offered to send a ferret down after it . . . or the vicar's daughter performing a Babinski response whose unthinking warning to the patient was that she was 'going to touch your sole . . .'

But while all this was going on, you were getting used to being with patients. And over the years, sixteen different doctors were giving you sixteen different takes on the sixteen different sorts of thing that crop up. And you learned stuff. You didn't realise it, but you did, and that's the best way.

Today, there's a mixture of tutorials and talks and tasters and Problem-Based Lounging and two or three bedside teaching sessions any of which you can miss out if you've got something else to do – like a part-time job at Tesco's.

Personally, I'd make the bedside teaching my priority.

---

133 OK – the initial assumption is he's picked up *a* book by accident.

PS For those adult doctors out there who think I've slipped up here in my attempt to make tips relevant to us too . . . just look at the tip title and think about it . . .

PPS They've also got hollow bones.

CAREER TIP 13: DON'T FOLLOW A WORD OF THE ADVICE IN THIS BOOK

13 Career Tips. Unlucky. We will follow the example of many hospitals who refuse to have a Ward 13 (ours is 12A) or a Bed 13 (ours is a fire-escape), and not include it in our ongoing count. But do not disregard the tip itself. Follow it implicitly (though this may result in some Dodgsonian dilemma).

Miscellaneous Tips

These are like, lots of different tips that, like don't fit perfectly into one of the other categories, like. Starting with like drugs like.

DRUG MANAGEMENT

DRUG MANAGEMENT TIP 1: IT TAKES THREE YEARS TO TREAT POLYMYALGIA RHEUMATICA

Actually three years and ten weeks.

At least.

Doctors make two major mistakes in the management of PMR. The first is to start prednisolone at too high a dose. If prednisolone 15 mg daily makes the disease disappear *as if by magic*, why would anyone start at 30 mg? Particularly since giving 30 mg loses the diagnostic confirmation that the resolution of symptoms *as if by magic* gives you (lots of different diseases will get a lot better on 30 mg, but only PMR will get better *as if by magic* on 15 mg). It's almost as if the connection of PMR with temporal arteritis – where you jump in with 30–40 mg prednisolone just in case the patient's about to wake up next morning blind in one eye – befuddles them into the reckless use of stupidly high doses against the desperate worry that otherwise the patient may wake up next morning . . . still with stiff shoulders.

The second mistake is arguably precipitated by the first. Nobody wants to be on 30 mg prednisolone for very long, so the dose is brought down quite sharpish every few days to 25 mg, 20 mg, 15 mg . . . and this sequence is continued . . . 10, 7.5, 5 . . . at which point *all the pains come back again*. And unfortunately in my experience once you lose control, very often the whole thing never quite works properly.

So what you should do is start lowish, and you reduce the dose ridiculously slowly. It goes like this:

15 mg	10 weeks
12.5 mg	6 weeks
10 mg	6 weeks
9 mg	6 weeks
8 mg	6 weeks
7.5 mg	6 weeks
7 mg	6 weeks
6.5 mg	6 weeks

. . . and so on, with half-mg decrements every six weeks.

Now, the mathematically astute, and smart-alec guys among you (girls won't have done this[134]) will have spotted that that's 24 × 6 weeks plus 10 weeks = 154 weeks = slightly *less* than three years. But nobody's really gonna remember to change every six weeks. Much better to change every 1.5 months, so every clinic visit I write down a 'template' for them to follow . . . *1st Jan – 10 mg, 15th Feb – 9 mg, 1st April – 8 mg, etc.* So it's 24 × 1.5 months plus ten weeks.

By following this slow reduction, patients maximise their chances of getting through to the end without a hitch. They'll be tempted to go faster, but persuade them not to. Tell them 7.5 mg prednisolone is pretty much what their own body normally makes steroid-wise . . . and side effects are very limited once they get down to that level . . . and they will get there quite quickly. I always tell them this, and it might even be true.

If aches come back a few days after a dose reduction, that's OK *as long as they all settle down before the next dose reduction is due*. Then you can go down the next step. If they don't settle, you go up one or (a maximum) two steps, get it back under control, then reduce even more slowly. You never (oops), ever (if you follow the plan) have to jump back up to 15 mg.

In answer to your questions.
1 Yes, weekly from the start in any older female. In males, I'd check a densitometry scan first to see if appropriate.

---

134 Again, because it's a waste of time, *not* because they ain't mathematically astute.

2 No. When they get OA pains or frozen shoulder pains you don't pretend it's the PMR coming back, and you don't up their steroid dosage.

3 What about it? You should only use it to help you with (2). My own theory is that steroids bring it down *per se*, so as the steroids are stopped it will naturally go up towards the normal for a person of that age.[135]

DRUG MANAGEMENT TIP 2: ODs AREN'T BD OR TDS

Theoretically, people who take overdoses are trying to kill themselves. Admittedly, in the real world it's more often a 'cry for help' – though clearly destined to fall on deaf ears since this particular real world is populated by hard-bitten doctors and harder-bitten nurses whose sole priority is to ensure you stay alive overnight (or at least until their shift finishes) rather than sort out all your personal and social problems of which they've got plenty enough of their own, thank you very much . . .

But whether it's a genuine cry for help or a cry for help, it's maybe too much to expect anyone going through either trauma to remember *exactly 'when did you take the tablets?'* But of course that's what we always ask them. Most of the time it's not particularly important, but there is that thing with the paracetamol.

I've always rated paracetamol overdose as a top diagnosis to look after since you get to use the word 'antidote' in all seriousness. People don't really do 'antidote' any more, but it was my favourite medical word from childhood days (certainly well ahead of 'kaolin poultice'). And paracetamol has actually got an antidote! So I take great pleasure in rhyming this off to all prospective antidotees – since all we need to tell us whether or not to use the antidote (see how seductive it is?) is the blood concentration of paracetamol, the time of the blood concentration and *exactly when did you take the tablets?*

But if a patient 'can't remember' in a mumbling voice because they were 'too drunk' (oooh . . . more chance they will need the antidote, as the level requiring antidote treatment is decreased) that puts the kybosh on the entire plan. Maybe.

Back in the old days, there wasn't much you could do other than take a guess whether or not to treat[136] since somehow, somebody, somewhere got it into their head that the antidote only worked properly in the first eight hours, patchily in the next four hours, after which it actually made things worse. The

135 All right then – it's 'what about the ESR?'
136 Seems a no-brainer. Treat, just in case. But what if the patient who does get the anaphylactic shock from the antidote does turn out to have taken exactly three paracetamol tablets?

weird thing was that we all swallowed this tosh since the proffered explanation *vis-à-vis* toxic and non-toxic metabolites and preferential pathways and stuff seemed to make sense and charmed the frontal cortexes[137] of young doctors in much the same way as long-term endowment policies. So there wasn't really time to perform the salutary manoeuvre of checking the blood paracetamol levels twice, and then draw the line between them, showing how fast the levels are dropping – and surmise the likely timing by fitting it onto the standard when-to-treat-paracetamol-poisoning graph which essentially outlines the normal decay of paracetamol levels – and Bob's your uncle.

The fitting-the-line part is a bit of a faff, but there is a quick way to get a yes/no answer on whether to treat. You take the standard graph, thus (*see* Figure 3).

You then get the first result (with no 'time-since' concept) and slap it on the treatment line ('1'). Then you mark the next blood result at the correct time *relative to the first result* ('2'). If this dot is above the line, treat.

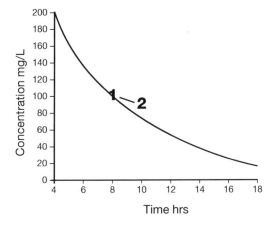

FIGURE 3 Paracetamol overdose

Predicting antidote requirements from two results of uncertain timing. In this case a result of 100 at unknown timing, with a result of 90 two hours later.

---

137 I know. But everybody seems to get befuddled when I mention 'Drug Kardices' so . . .

(How long should you wait before doing the second level? Not known. Maybe because this is a personal, anecdotal-type tip. It's like . . . long enough to be able to draw a sensible line, within the limits of the reliability of your assay. Maybe two hours? As I say, it depends on your assay. My own theory is that the shortest time possible to get the junior to do a blood test and then do another one should be time enough . . . And I should mention that I invoke this tip only when the decision has been made to NOT treat – to give an extra chance to get it right. I don't delay treatment where otherwise it would have been given.)

DRUG MANAGEMENT TIP 2a: TO BE USED IN CONJUNCTION WITH DRUG MANAGEMENT TIP 2

The antidote is N-acetyl cysteine.

DRUG MANAGEMENT TIP 3: ALTER PHENYTOIN DOSAGE CAREFULLY

There's a story about the best way to get drunk at a party – as told by clinical pharmacologists (not actually told *at* parties since, as outlined elsewhere, clinical pharmacologists do not get invited to such things).

The start of the plan is to drink the alcoholic beverage of your choice reasonably rapidly[138] until just nicely tipsy. Thereafter you drink at a steady one-unit-alcohol-per-hour as, the theory has it, most people's metabolism when fully up-and-running will break down one unit of alcohol per hour – so you can stay at that nicely-tipsy state. Any faster, and the extra alcohol will accumulate and you'll get hammered.

You might think from this that if you drink ¾ of a unit per hour from the start, then you'll pretty much never have any alcohol in your system. But that unit-per-hour is the *peak* rate. If you are drinking less and your blood levels are less, your enzymes don't work so hard, and you'll still get a bit tiddly.

So what's this all got to do with phenytoin? Well, the hourly alcohol story is a bit like the daily phenytoin story. Whilst your system gradually increases its efforts to metabolise phenytoin as the dosage increases, there quite quickly comes a point where its efforts reach a plateau – and the concentration at this point is approximately where phenytoin actually starts to work. The

---

138 . . . as opposed to 'as rapidly as possible before leaving the house to avoid having to actually buy the stuff yourself instead of taking dad's . . .'

pharmacology chaps like to talk about a changeover from First-Order to Zero-Order kinetics ('saturation kinetics') and stuff like that, but the bottom line is that even small increases in dosage above this level will cause disproportion-ately large increases in blood phenytoin levels. You can get the idea from a graph of the 'steady-state' blood phenytoin vs. daily dosage for a Mr John Doe (*see* Figure 4).

So Dr Doh, who doesn't know this concept, might look at a blood level of 10 mg/L when Mr Doe is taking 300 mg of phenytoin per day and think 'we'd like that level to be 15 mg/L,[139] so I'll give him a 50% rise in dose to 450 mg per day.' A quick look at the chart shows where that would put the patient (in hospital, probably) once the drug reaches its 'steady-state' (classically in five half-lives' time – around 5–7 days in the case of phenytoin, which does at least give Dr Doh a chance to read a medical book, check with a colleague, or leave the country).

Once phenytoin levels get up anywhere near the 'target range', you should increase only in 25 mg increments. The same goes for reducing the dose when

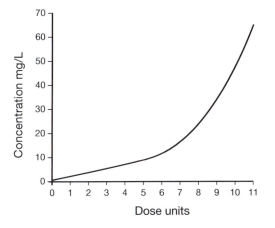

FIGURE 4 Phenytoin concentration vs. dosage

---

139 Middle of 'target range'. But only if the epilepsy is not already controlled. Blood levels are not as important as clinical state.

you think the patient's levels are a bit high. Halving the dose will almost certainly bring levels down to negligible (unless the previous physician was a total tube) so after a missing out a dose or two, a reduction by 25 mg or 50 mg is almost always adequate.

DRUG MANAGEMENT TIP 4: PATIENTS DON'T REALLY NEED FERROUS SULPHATE 200 mg TDS

No clinical evidence for this tip.

But the maths is enough for me.

Men need to absorb 1 mg of iron per day. Women (because of the menses) need 2 mg per day. We absorb approximately 10% of the iron we ingest (as it happens, the % increases if we become iron deficient) so we need 10–20 mg iron per day in our diet.

If you become iron deficient for any of the usual reasons (blood loss, poor diet, etc.[140]) there is no conceivable reason why you would want to throw 600 mg per day at the problem – a manoeuvre which can often be counter-productive since a large number of people will get either constipation or diarrhoea (spookily enough) on full-dose iron and will stop taking the tablets. My suggestion would be one tablet per day – 200 mg is ample – and if you have to take them for longer, so be it.

DRUG MANAGEMENT TIP 5: TREAT THE PATIENT'S THYROID, NOT THE POPULATION'S

Thyroid Stimulating Hormone (TSH) is produced somewhere in the brain (I think it's the anterior pituitary) when somewhere else in the brain (I think it's the hypothalamus) decides the body needs more thyroid hormone (thyroxine) floating about. TSH tells somewhere in the neck (I'm pretty sure that one's the thyroid gland) to make more thyroxine. That's why, as somebody drifts towards primary hypothyroidism (i.e. the thyroid itself failing) their TSH keeps getting higher and higher, 'imploring the thyroid to exert itself' as they don't quite say in *Peter Rabbit*. The over-flogged thyroid just manages to keep thyroxine in the 'low–normal range' until finally it packs in completely and we get the low-thyroxine/high-TSH pattern of primary hypothyroidism.

---

140 Very occasionally poor absorption might be the primary problem – but that's a totally different and rare ball game (let's call it . . . *pelota*). If you know about it, they may need parenteral iron. If you don't, low-dose iron might help you spot the rarity.

So.

If you treat this with thyroxine, and the patient's thyroxine comes up to 'normal', but the TSH is still high, that means the patient's body wants more thyroxine made. *This* 'normal' isn't *their* normal (which makes sense since it's just a range in which 95% tend to have their thyroid levels). So in a treated hypothyroid patient where the thyroxine level is normal, but TSH is high, you should give them just a bit more thyroxine.

And you can take it a bit further. If the TSH is slap-dab in the middle of the 'normal' range, but they still have hypothyroid symptoms, even if thyroxine is at a highish level . . . then you can still try a small increase in thyroxine dosage. This is a population normal, not necessarily theirs: bring *their* TSH down into the low normal – maybe that's where it usually sits. Maybe it's actually *up* to persuade their thyroid to make more hormone, which it can't do, so you have to give it in tablet form. Worth a try.

Note, this is for patients on thyroxine already. Not those not on thyroxine who insist they must have hypothyroidism despite the absolutely normal tests and lack of clinical signs because it says in *Red Mariepolitan* magazine that . . .

DRUG MANAGEMENT TIP 6: WARFARIN TAKES A COUPLE OF DAYS TO KICK IN

Let's say it's Monday.

A patient comes in with an unconnected (or indeed connected) illness and the resident/JHO/PRHO/SPV/FY1[141] notices they're on warfarin 3 mg, and checks the INR. It's 1.5.[142] The SHO/Reg/ST2/SDF knows it should be around 2.5, so the warfarin is increased to 4 mg.

Tuesday, the INR is 1.6. Clearly the increase wasn't enough so the warfarin that evening goes to 5 mg.

Wednesday's INR is 1.9 so the warfarin is increased to 6 mg.

On Thursday, the INR is 2.5. Everybody's happy, the patient goes home and all's right with the world – except that the INR of 2.5 reflects the increase to 4 mg from two nights earlier beginning to kick in, and she's toddling off home on 6 mg.

Everybody knows it takes a couple of days for the new dose of warfarin to have its effect, but conveniently forgets this since otherwise everything

---

141 Might have got carried away there. I think one of those is Captain Scarlet's car.
142 Sometimes I gratuitously ask the junior what the units are, just to watch them sweat – 'cos there aren't any 'cos it's a ratio (vs. normal). Doesn't mean I'm a bad person.

just seems to take too long. It's also a bit counter-intuitive. So if you do have trouble with the mental phase-shift, try this:

Pretend that today's result is the result from two days ago, and see if what you just did with the dosage makes any sense at all.

STATISTICS TIPS

We should all have some basic idea of statistics – if only because it's fun picking holes in people's strongly held convictions so you can win arguments, even when they're right.

STATISTICS TIP 1: UNDERSTAND THE POWER GAME

The Power Game is played in many echelons of the NHS. Particularly in the 'drug procurement' areas of NICE, SMC, major Drugs and Therapeutics Committees, etc. Surprisingly often you'll hear people in these upper echelons, when faced with a surprise positive finding in a drug trial, come out with the 'was the trial powered for that?' canard.

It really doesn't matter.

If you get a significant finding in a trial, it doesn't matter whether it was 'powered' to find that out. It's still a positive finding. Power only matters if you *fail* to show any difference, e.g. between two treatments – then it is important to see if your trial was well-enough designed, had enough patients, clear enough targets . . . , i.e. was *powered* to find the difference if it was there.

As an example, you invent a new antibiotic and you design a trial using 20 patients with pneumonia – 10 get the drug, 10 don't – and you take note of exactly how many die in each group (always good to keep outcomes simple). Arguably the most underpowered trial since Adam 'proved' that you should never do what a woman tells you. No way enough patients. Chances are nobody (or almost nobody . . .) will die in either group, leaving you back where you started. But let's say you happen to do this just at the start of a mini-epidemic of the most virulent pneumonia ever to hit the planet. All 10 patients in your placebo group die. All 10 in your drug group survive. A hugely statistically significant difference. This drug works! You may have been 'lucky'[143] to prove it – but it is still proven (as much as stats ever prove

---

143 Lucky enough to end up in jail if you indeed used an inactive placebo.

anything). Small trials often overestimate the extent of a drug's value (the serendipity helping them get the p-value), but the finding that an effect exists remains genuine.

Alternatively, let's say two patients in the placebo group die, but none in the drug group. Since two such events would occur in the same group by chance half of the time, this is no way significant. Even if there were three deaths to none – still not significant. But this would NOT prove that the drug *doesn't* work. Indeed the results are suspicious that it might. This time we do look at the power as we have failed to prove a difference and indeed we see that the trial is hugely underpowered to show a difference that might be there. So this needs a bigger (better) trial.

We'll not go through the actual formula for calculation of power, as I'd have to look it up and that would go against the ethos of this book as well as taking me a few minutes. However, it helps to know it includes such things as:

1 Number of subjects in study. More subjects, more power (easier to prove that men are taller than women with 1000 in each group than with five).

2 Standard deviation of the thing you are measuring. Less variation, more power (easier to prove which of two classes of schoolchildren is the older, than two disparate groups of random humans . . . say, two railway carriages of people. If we took six kids from each class, it'd be obvious; six people from each carriage, however . . .).

3 Expected level of difference between the two groups. Bigger difference, more power (easier to prove 25-year-old men are taller than 3-year-olds than than[144] 15-year-olds).

4 How 'significant' you require results to be. Less significance required, more powerful (easier to not-really prove something). Not the *best* way to increase the power.

So the power might be 'an 80% chance of proving at the $p<0.05$ level a difference in height between the groups (when it's expected to be about 5 cm)'. Such calculations are usually made before a study – at the design stage. The last three are factored in to give an answer as to how many subjects (Factor 1) would be required to give decent power.

So Adam's right then.

---

144 So why the squiggly red lines?

STATISTICS TIP 2: PICK A CARD . . . ANY CARD . . . TRY AGAIN! . . .

What the person at the top of the previous tip really wanted to know was: *is this 'surprise' a genuine finding or just an incidental when they were looking at so many things and doing so many 'tests' that one of them just happened to be significant?*

We all know the concept. The basic assumption in statistics to us lay-person types is that a p-value of <0.05 is 'significant'. This result would happen by chance less than 0.05 of the time (i.e. less than 0.05 out of 1, i.e. less than 5% of the time, i.e. less than one time in twenty[145]). We are happy to accept that level as reasonably unlikely so there must be some significant factor in play. More properly, the assumption is that if you predict something will happen (*see* Statistics Tip 3) and do a study where that something does indeed happen, and you show that the possibility of this happening entirely by chance is less than 5% – then you can take the reasoning behind your prediction as 'proven'.

(Adam should really have asked a whole bunch of women whether he should eat the apple. Not necessarily 20 other women. It's like tossing a coin. Heads/Tails. Yes/No. The first heads is a one-in-two chance. Two heads = 1/4. Three heads 1/8. Four heads 1/16. Five heads 1/32. So five heads is a less than one-in-twenty chance – if you suspect a double-headed coin, five heads 'proves' it[146] and you shouldn't do what the wife tells you.)

But if you do lots of tests, you will randomly throw up the occasional one-in-twenty chance. We often think of this as 'do twenty tests and one of them will be a one-in-twenty chance.' It isn't as simple as that. If you pick a card from the pack, there's a one-in-four chance it'll be a heart. That doesn't mean if you pick four cards you'll always get one heart. You might get none, you might get two . . . three . . . four. This is one reason why the Bonferroni correction – where you multiply your p-value by the number of tests you've done (e.g. if you do four tests, a p=0.025 would become p=0.1 and 'lose' its 'significance') is an over-glib attempt to solve this problem, making the criteria too stringent.

There's no simple mathematical way to be precise about the effect of multiple tests. It is perhaps enough to be aware of the problem and view any moderately 'significant' findings picked up in such a way (either by yourself or in others' work) as something requiring further study, but not necessarily proving anything.

---

145 Not 20–1, but 19–1. Not vital here, but more important down at the lower figures and down at the bookies.

146 Assuming you knew/suspected it was double-headed. *See* Statistics Tip 3.

STATISTICS TIP 3: IGNORE INDEX CASES

So I'm at this conference and this ginger-haired guy's presentation shows: 20% of patients with Disease A will previously have had Disease B – so they must be linked.

And I ask why they looked for this bizarre connection, and it's because they happened to notice three of their patients with rareish Disease A had previously had rareish Disease B so they looked at their whole population.

And I ask if they included their first three 'index' cases . . . and he says . . . 'Yes. Someone told us that we shouldn't do that, but I don't see what the problem is . . .'

Interesting.

It went something like this. They'd got their first three patients – then out of the next 17 cases of Disease A, one had previously had Disease B. Put them together and you get 4 out of 20. 20%! As long as you ignore the good advice: ignore the index cases.

This isn't really a tip. It's a rule.

In the world-sized world of medicine, lots of things will happen by chance. If you notice one of these things and think it may not be by chance, you quite rightly should study this – by starting from scratch. Look at lots of new cases and see if you can prove your theory. In the above example, the best estimate for the Diseases A and B association is 1 in 17, not 4 in 20. 6% rather than 20%.

We can go back to our double-headed coin in the last tip. If we specifically suspect a double-headed coin, then five consecutive heads 'prove' a bogus fourpenny piece at the $p<0.05$ level. If, however, we suspect a bogus coin – either double-headed or double-tailed – then the first throw doesn't count except to give us an index case. For example, we throw a 'tail'. We now suspect this is a two-tailed coin[147] and the next five throws might 'prove' this. Five heads would not now prove a double-headed coin. To use a longer-odds starter – if someone told you a die[148] was fixed to come up six every time and your first two throws were a six – that would be very suspicious (1:36). If they just said it was fixed in some way and your first two throws were both threes – that's less so (1:6).

Alternatively let's use the Bonferroni too-many-tests concept – using 100 coins to represent 'the world'. We toss them all. Fifty heads (unlikely

---

147 Not a reference to 'two-tailed significance tests' which concern the tails of a Gaussian distribution, yet spookily having *exactly the same effect* on the stats.

148 If anyone ever complains you're being pedantic using this singular, ask them if they'd ever say 'the dice is cast'.

– but let's not get into that). Toss those fifty . . . 25 heads. Toss those 25 . . . 12 heads. Toss those 12 . . . 6 heads. We now have six coins that have come up heads four times in a row. Toss them again – is anything that turns up heads a bogus coin? Obviously not. But say we hadn't made it so obvious by tossing only the heads coins again. Say we toss all 100 coins the four times. And our ginger-haired guy[149] has been watching closely and is standing near one of our four-headers. He picks it up, and tosses it once more . . .

FROM THE 'OTHER SIDE' TIPS

My writing of this book was interrupted by an excuse for me to spend some time as a patient (well, it's better than doing rheumatology clinics). This prompted me to include a few tips about seeing things from the patient's point of view.

OTHER-SIDE TIP 1: SOMEHOW . . . FIND OUT WHAT IT'S LIKE

Seems a bit bizarre. Like I'm suggesting you go get sick or something. But somehow, someway, you should try to get a taste of it. I'd always felt I had some insight into the 'other side' – having had a couple of proper childhood illnesses with hospital stays – but recent experience reminded me that things are different as an adult (not sure I'd now tolerate a grown man swinging a leather belt ['tawse'] as hard as he could at my unprotected hand[150]) as well as memory being fickle. Patients *do* have a miserable time in hospital, including:

1 Food – much worse than I'd ever thought. My concept was of just-a-bit-worse-than-canteen-food, but that totally failed to pick up on its complete awfulness. It is simply inedible. Often cooked miles away and hours earlier (on Friday, I knew it was fried fish for lunch after I smelled its arrival in the building at 9.30 am), the sort of food we throw up at patients (cut out the middleman?) must surely slow down recovery. So if one of them is having food brought in from outside, it doesn't mean they're posh or picky or awkward. Just human. So don't give 'em a bad time.

---

149 Nothing against ginger hair. They're not a bunch of people who throw coins all the time (whatever that would be). Just an adapted cinematic device so you immediately know who I mean. (Cf. glasses on wife in *Strangers on a Train*, the girl's red coat in *Schindler's List*, Hitler's moustache . . .)

150 On re-reading, I should clarify this is a reference to schooldays. Glasgow paediatricians used a stick.

2 Drug rounds – I've always filled in timings for drugs based on my simple grasp of maths and my even simpler grasp of pharmacokinetics. What it means to the patient doesn't occur to me – until it's eleven o'clock at night and I'm desperately wanting to sleep and I've only now just been given my night-time medicines which include diclofenac (yes it *does* give me heartburn/reflux, as it happens . . . and I *am* on anticoagulants at the moment) and lactulose (which gives *everybody* heartburn and was described perfectly by a nursing colleague as like being given 'someone else's saliva to drink') which between them will burn my chest to a frazzle the second my angle-of-recumbency goes below 50° (Tip 1 for in-patients is *learn how to sleep upright*). So, just for fun, try a bit of thought-process next time you're writing up the times for drug dosing.

3 Ward rounds – maybe it's just me, but I felt the day was not 'my own' until the doctors[151] had been to see me. So I delayed washing, shaving, phoning my bookmaker, etc. till later in case I missed them. So doing a ward round when expected, and no later than necessary, suddenly makes sense to me.

4 Dissociation – one unnerving aspect of being a patient is the realisation that the people coming in to see you . . . doctors, nurses, relatives . . . have all got 'proper' lives going on, whilst you are stuck there. If this is emphasised by a group of, e.g. doctors sharing a laugh over last night's curry, Sunday's football or other liveliness which no way could involve your battered body, it can become irritating. Of course I like a bit of banter on the ward round – same as everywhere else – but you should make sure that the patient feels he/she is part of the fun (certainly rather than any butt). I'll often repeat for the benefit of the patient what one of the juniors has said at the case trolley (since only if it's confidential medical info will they have already shouted it out to the entire ward) if the rest of us have responded with laughter – if it was really funny, I'll pretend it was me. Amongst other things, it does reassure the patient that it wasn't at their expense. And lets them know *whose side we're on*.

   (Before you get confused about which side we *are* on: when we're diagnosing 'tricky' patients it's *us against them*, when we're getting the properly sick ones better it's *us-and-them against the world*.)

5 Platitudes – if a patient has a problem or worry, don't just say 'it'll be fine'. Tell them what you think is causing it, whether you need to do anything specific about it, and *why* it'll (probably) be fine.

---

151 I say 'doctors', but as a consultant I was studiously avoided by anyone themselves below the level of prime minister – leaving my exposure to medical staff quirkily limited to one five-minute contact per day.

So go get sick or something. Or at least be aware of what it's like, and allow for your patient's apparent idiosyncrasies accordingly.

OTHER-SIDE TIP 2: IF YOU ARE ON THE OTHER SIDE, THERE'S NO FOOLPROOF APPROACH

We all know there is a doctor-as-patient problem – quoted by the anti-doctor brigade (that's everyone who isn't themself a doctor) as due to 'not being in control any more' and by the pro-doctor brigade (doctors) as due to 'knowing too much'. Not surprisingly, I fall in the latter camp. When you know what side effects drugs can cause, and what things can go wrong with various proce-dures, it is nigh impossible to face the slightest manoeuvre with equanimity.

Before my recent admission, the advice from my Clinical Nurse Specialist was to 'do what I was told' (though less abrupt) and I agreed. Let the guys who know what they're doing, do what they do best. Don't try to second-guess. But next day the other CNS said 'don't be afraid to speak up'.

So who's right?

Who's *always* right?

Both of them. Neither. Nobody.

Just like everything else, the doctor-as-patient scenario can only be dealt with on a case-by-case basis. Indeed an event-by-event basis. Sometimes you need to go with the flow, other times you have to speak up and get things changed. Simple. The only problem is . . . *you will always get these round the wrong way*.

Ergo:

➤ If you think your epidural's a bit *high*, you'll say nothing, and get lots of low pain.

➤ If you hear nurses playing around with aforementioned epidural, you'll say something ('how about wearing some sterile mittens!'[152]) and they'll point out they're nowhere near the spinal site, and you'll feel a right toffee.

➤ If your IV drug dosage sounds quadruple what you'd use, you'll say nothing and *skaboooooosh!*

➤ If your IV drug dosage sounds a quarter what you'd use, you'll say something ('that won't be enough'), they'll listen to you and *skaboooooosh!*

➤ If they're just anaesthetising you and you think you hear somebody saying it's your *right* kidney they're going for and . . . you're . . . sure . . . . . . tha . . .

---

152 'Cos you don't want your spinal fluid smelling of chips.

OTHER-SIDE TIP 3: PICK AN IDIOSYNCRATIC FORMAT (YOU LIKE!) FOR YOUR TEA/COFFEE

The first time I was asked in the ward how I liked my tea, I told them a tiny bit of milk and *one-third-of-a-teaspoonful* of sugar.

This was deservedly slagged off as being a bit control-freakish.

The second time I was asked, I told them the same.

This was also deservedly slagged off.

The third time, they didn't need to ask, as they all knew and remembered this slag-offable choice.

OK. I get a totally undeserved reputation as a pernickety blighter, but all the subsequent times I get tea – without their having to ask or getting it all wrong or me having to trouble them – it's how I quite like it (though it would have been better with four-elevenths of a spoonful).

PS Cardiology guru thinks this tip isn't important enough, but what's more critical to recovery than a good cup of tea?

SURVIVAL/CAREER TIPS

SURVIVAL/CAREER TIP 1: MAKE *NEVER* SURE *TAKE* YOU *A* HAVE *LUNCH* BIG *BREAK* LUNCH *AT* BREAKS *ALL*

SURVIVAL	CAREER
1 Taking time over eating is good for your digestion.	*You'll get more work done.*
2 Taking a proper break from the morning stresses of medicine will 'recharge your batteries' (sorry) and help you cope with the afternoon stresses.	*People will think you seriously want to be a manager.*
3 Discussing patients with colleagues in an informal scenario gives a chance to 'brainstorm' in a way perhaps inappropriate with formal referrals.	
4 Discussing football, golf, art, TV, films, books, philosophy with your colleagues can foster better relationships.	
5 All the things in 4 also help achieve the target in 2.	
6 Problems with rotas, cover, juniors, seniors, can be teased out in a friendly manner.	
7 You'll live longer.	…mmmm…tricky…

PUBLISHING TIPS

TIP 101: DON'T CALL YOUR BOOK *100 TOP TIPS*

One hundred and one sounds a lot cooler, and it makes people think they're getting some sort of bargain.

Appendix 1: Answers

1 Inferior
2 Inferior
3 Mobitz
4 Wenckebach
5 Ventricular

Appendix 2: Culprits

JA	Dr Jacqueline Adams. Cardiologist, Victoria Infirmary, Glasgow.
HD	Dr Helen Dallal. Gastroenterologist, North Tees Trust.
JH	Dr John Hinnie. Endocrinologist, Victoria Infirmary, Glasgow.
IL	Dr Iain Lennox. Department of Medicine for the Elderly, Victoria Infirmary, Glasgow.
HMcA	Dr Howard McAlpine. Cardiologist, Victoria Infirmary, Glasgow.
DR	Dr David Raeside. Respiratory Physician, Victoria Infirmary, Glasgow.
SDS	Dr Stefan Slater. Endocrinologist (retired . . . mainly), Glasgow and Edinburgh.
CW	Dr Caroline Whitton. Department of Medicine for the Elderly, Victoria Infirmary, Glasgow.

Index